Whole Body Menopause Guide

Holistic and Evidence-Based Approach to
Balance Hormones, Counteract Weight
Gain, Cope with Mood Swings, Manage
Hot Flashes, Minimize Night Sweats,
and Sleep Better

Michele Altobello, BSN, RN, AMB-BC

Table of Contents

Introduction

At the age of 40, I found myself sitting in yet another doctor's office, trying to make sense of the whirlwind of changes my body was experiencing. Hot flashes, night sweats, mood swings, and unrelenting fatigue had become my unwelcome companions. Yet, each time I sought help, I was met with the same dismissive response: "You're too young for menopause." The tests I asked for were always denied. It felt like an uphill battle, struggling alone with symptoms that were all too real.

It wasn't until I took matters into my own hands that I began to understand what was happening to me. After years of suffering, I sought an evaluation from a nurse practitioner, who ordered the necessary testing and ultimately diagnosed me with premature menopause. This realization was both a relief and a challenge—a relief because I finally had a name for what I was experiencing and a challenge because I had been on my own so far, with limited guidance and support.

Allow me to introduce myself. My name is Michele Altobello, and I am a board-certified registered nurse with more than 20 years of experience. I have also walked the path you are on.

Managing menopause requires a holistic approach. This means addressing the whole body, not just individual symptoms. In this book, you will find chapters dedicated to symptom relief, along with detailed discussions on each body system affected by menopause. Each chapter will provide you with symptoms to watch for, strategies to reduce those symptoms, and various treatment options. We will examine the most current holistic and medical perspectives and discuss hormone replacement and other evidence-based resources. Each section contains practical advice, exercises, and treatment options you can apply daily. A well-rounded approach ensures you find what works best for your unique situation.

One of this book's key, critical goals is to empower you. Menopause is not simply something to endure; it is a phase of life in which you can thrive. Many women have walked this path, and with the right tools and knowledge, you will have the strength to navigate this phase and improve your quality of life. After reading this book, you will know that you are not alone on this journey.

Chapter 1:

Understanding Menopause

By the time I was diagnosed with premature menopause, my symptoms were overwhelming—hot flashes, night sweats, and mood swings had taken over my life. Receiving validation that my symptoms were genuine and not merely a figment of my imagination helped me to understand the changes my body was going through. This chapter aims to provide you with that same understanding. By knowing what menopause is and what to expect, you can take control of your health and well-being.

What Is Menopause?

Menopause marks the end of menstrual cycles and is diagnosed after 12 consecutive months without a period. This natural biological process signifies the end of your reproductive years. The average age of onset is around 51, but it can start in your 40s or even late 50s. The timing varies widely among women and is influenced by genetics, lifestyle, and overall health.

Natural menopause occurs gradually. Your ovaries begin to produce fewer hormones, particularly estrogen and progesterone, leading to the cessation of menstruation. This decline in hormone production affects various bodily functions, causing the symptoms commonly associated with menopause.

Hot flashes, night sweats, and mood swings are some of the most well-known symptoms, but there are many others, including sleep disturbances, weight gain, and changes in sexual health.

In some cases, medical interventions can inadvertently induce menopause. Surgical menopause occurs when the ovaries are removed, often due to conditions such as ovarian cancer or endometriosis. This abrupt removal of the ovaries leads to an immediate drop in hormone levels, causing sudden onset of menopausal symptoms. Medical menopause can also be induced by treatments such as chemotherapy or radiation therapy, which can damage the ovaries and reduce hormone production.

You need to understand the differences between natural and induced menopause to manage your symptoms effectively. Natural menopause allows for a gradual transition, giving your body time to adjust to the hormonal changes. In contrast, induced menopause leads to immediate and often more severe symptoms, requiring a more aggressive approach to symptom management.

The clinical criteria for diagnosing menopause are straightforward but essential. You are considered to have reached menopause if you have not had a menstrual period for 12 consecutive months—and no other underlying medical conditions are causing this absence. This definition helps healthcare providers determine the appropriate action for managing your symptoms and overall health.

One of the first steps in understanding menopause is recognizing that it is a natural part of aging. It is not a disease or a condition that needs to be cured but a phase of life that requires adjustment and management. By learning about the changes happening in your body, you can make informed decisions about your health and well-being.

The variation in the age of onset and the intensity of symptoms can be attributed to several factors. Genetics plays a significant role. If your mother or sisters experienced early menopause, you might, too. Lifestyle factors such as smoking, diet, and physical activity also influence the timing and severity of menopause. Women who smoke typically experience menopause earlier than nonsmokers. A healthy diet and regular exercise can help mitigate some of the symptoms.

Understanding menopause also involves acknowledging its emotional and psychological impact. The hormonal fluctuations can affect your mood, leading to feelings of sadness, anxiety, or irritability. These emotional changes are a normal part of the process but can be challenging to manage. Seeking support from healthcare providers, mental health professionals, or support groups can make a significant difference in your emotional well-being.

Menopause is a unique experience for every woman. No two experiences are exactly alike; what works for one person may not work for another. Keep reading to learn about various options and strategies that can help you manage your symptoms effectively. From hormone replacement therapy to holistic treatments, you will find a wealth of information to help you throughout this phase of life.

The Stages of Menopause: Perimenopause, Menopause, and Postmenopause

Perimenopause

Perimenopause is the transitional phase leading up to menopause. It typically begins in your late 40s, but it starts earlier for some. This stage is marked by hormonal fluctuations that can cause various symptoms. You might notice irregular menstrual cycles, where your periods become less predictable. In some months, they might be heavy, and in other months, they might be light or even absent. These changes are a direct result of your ovaries producing varying levels of estrogen and progesterone.

During perimenopause, you might experience the onset of symptoms such as hot flashes and sleep disturbances. Hot flashes can feel like sudden waves of heat that spread throughout your body, causing sweating and discomfort. They can happen at any time, often disrupting your daily activities. Sleep disturbances are also common. You might find it difficult to fall asleep, or you might wake up frequently at night. These symptoms can be frustrating and exhausting, but knowing they are a normal part of perimenopause will help you manage them better.

Menopause

The transition from perimenopause to menopause is a significant phase. Menopause is officially diagnosed when you have gone 12 consecutive months without a menstrual period. The average age for this transition is around 51, though it can vary. During this time, your ovaries have stopped releasing eggs, and your body produces much lower levels of estrogen and progesterone. This hormonal shift can bring about a range of symptoms, including mood swings, weight gain, and changes in sexual health. You might notice a decrease in libido or experience vaginal dryness, making intercourse uncomfortable.

It's also important to differentiate between early menopause and premature menopause. Early menopause occurs between the ages of 40 and 45, whereas premature menopause happens before the age of 40. Various factors can cause early or premature menopause, including genetics, autoimmune disorders, and medical treatments such as chemotherapy. If you experience symptoms of menopause before age 40, you need to consult a healthcare provider to determine the cause and appropriate management strategies.

One of menopause's most significant impacts is on fertility and reproductive health. Once you reach menopause, you are unable to conceive naturally. This time of life can be emotional, especially if you had hoped to have more children. Understanding and accepting this change is crucial for moving forward. If your feelings become overwhelming, discuss them with a healthcare provider or a counselor.

Postmenopause

Postmenopause is the phase that follows menopause and lasts for the rest of your life. Once you have been without a period for a year, you are considered post-menopausal. Some symptoms, like hot flashes and night sweats, might continue during this time, but they often become less intense. However, the decrease in estrogen can lead to other long-term health concerns. You are at a higher risk for osteoporosis, as lower estrogen levels can result in decreased bone density, making bones more fragile and prone to fractures. Cardiovascular diseases also become more of a concern. Estrogen has a protective effect on the heart, and its decline can increase the risk of heart disease and stroke.

Long-term health monitoring becomes critical in postmenopause. Regular checkups with your healthcare provider can help catch and manage conditions like osteoporosis and cardiovascular diseases early. Bone-density scans and cholesterol tests are essential tools for monitoring your health. Lifestyle changes, including maintaining a balanced diet rich in calcium and vitamin D, engaging in regular physical activity, and avoiding smoking and excessive alcohol, can help you manage these risks.

The timeline and duration of each menopause stage varies widely among women. Perimenopause can last for several years, often between three and seven, but it can be shorter or longer.

Understanding these stages and what to expect at each phase can empower you to take proactive steps in managing your health. Each stage of menopause brings challenges and changes, but with the proper knowledge and support, you can navigate them with confidence.

Hormonal Changes During Menopause

Estrogen is a critical hormone in the female body; it plays an important role in various systems. During your reproductive years, estrogen regulates the menstrual cycle, maintains bone density, supports cardiovascular health, and influences the skin's elasticity and moisture levels. As menopause approaches, the decline in estrogen levels triggers a cascade of changes. One of the first and most noticeable symptoms is vaginal dryness. This occurs because estrogen helps maintain the thickness and elasticity of vaginal tissues, along with natural lubrication. Without sufficient estrogen, these tissues become thinner and less elastic, leading to discomfort and dryness. Another common symptom is hot flashes. These sudden waves of heat can be intense and disruptive. The part of the brain that regulates body temperature is called the hypothalamus, and during menopause, it becomes more sensitive to temperature changes due to lower estrogen levels.

Progesterone, another critical hormone, also sees a decline during menopause. During your reproductive years, progesterone helps regulate the menstrual cycle and prepare the uterus for pregnancy. Its decline is most evident in perimenopause when irregular menstrual cycles become common. Progesterone's role in maintaining pregnancy means its reduction can also affect your mood and sleep patterns. The balance between estrogen and progesterone is delicate, and when this balance is disrupted, it can lead to various symptoms, including mood swings, anxiety, and sleep disturbances. Testosterone, though often associated with men, is also present in women and plays a role in maintaining libido and muscle mass. During menopause, testosterone levels can decline, leading to a decrease in sexual desire and potentially contributing to the loss of muscle mass and strength.

Hormonal imbalances during menopause are responsible for many of the symptoms you may experience. These imbalances can manifest in various ways, from the physical to the emotional. Mood swings are a common symptom, often leaving you feeling irritable or anxious without an apparent reason. Weight gain, particularly around the abdomen, is another frequent issue. This is partly due to the reduction in estrogen, which affects how your body stores fat. Maintaining hormonal balance through diet and lifestyle becomes paramount. A diet rich in phytoestrogens, found in foods like soy and flaxseeds, can help. Regular exercise not only helps manage weight but also boosts mood and energy levels. For some, hormone replacement therapy (HRT) may be an option to consider. HRT can help replenish estrogen and progesterone levels, alleviating many symptoms of hormonal imbalance.

Menopause and the Endocrine System

Menopause doesn't just affect the primary sex hormones; it has a broader impact on the entire endocrine system. The thyroid gland, which regulates metabolism, can be particularly affected. Thyroid hormones and estrogen interact closely, so fluctuations in estrogen can lead to thyroid imbalances. Symptoms of thyroid dysfunction, such as fatigue, weight changes, and mood disturbances, can overlap with menopausal symptoms, making diagnosis and management more complex. Adrenal glands, responsible for producing stress hormones like cortisol, also come into play. During menopause, your adrenal glands may compensate for the declining sex hormones by increasing cortisol production, which can lead to increased stress levels and fatigue, further complicating the menopausal experience.

Research has shown that estrogen activity in the brain changes during menopause. A study conducted by Weill Cornell Medicine (2024) used PET imaging to observe estrogen receptor density in the brains of women aged 40–65. The study found that post-menopausal and premenopausal women had higher estrogen receptor densities in specific brain regions compared to premenopausal women. This increase is thought to be a compensatory response to the drop in estrogen levels, affecting cognitive and mood symptoms. High receptor density in cognitive regions like the hippocampus was associated with lower scores on cognitive tests. In contrast, higher densities in areas like the thalamus were linked to mood symptoms, such as depression. This research underscores the complex relationship between estrogen and brain function during menopause, highlighting the importance of hormonal balance for mental well-being.

Understanding the hormonal changes during menopause can empower you to take control of your symptoms. By recognizing the roles of estrogen, progesterone, and testosterone and how their imbalances affect your body, you can make informed decisions about your health.

The Role of Genetics and Lifestyle in Menopause

Genetic factors can heavily influence the timing and experience of menopause. If your mother or sisters experienced early menopause, there's a higher likelihood that you might, too. Family history can provide valuable clues about your menopausal timeline. Recent studies have identified hundreds of genetic variants that influence the age at which menopause occurs. These genetic markers can explain why some women start menopause in their early 40s while others don't experience it until their late 50s. Genetic predisposition also affects the severity and types of symptoms you might encounter. For instance, if your family has a history of severe hot flashes or mood swings during menopause, you might be more likely to experience similar symptoms.

Lifestyle choices play a crucial role in how menopause manifests and progresses. Diet and exercise are significant factors that can either alleviate or exacerbate symptoms. A balanced diet rich in fruits, vegetables, whole grains, and lean proteins can help manage weight gain, stabilize mood, and improve overall energy levels. Regular exercise, including aerobic activities and strength training, can reduce the frequency and severity of hot flashes, improve sleep quality, and boost mental well-being. Exercise also supports cardiovascular health, which is particularly important as the risk of heart disease increases post-menopause.

The Importance of Stress Management

Stress management is another essential part of menopausal health. Chronic stress can exacerbate hormonal imbalances, leading to more severe symptoms. Techniques such as yoga, meditation, and deep-breathing exercises can help you maintain hormonal balance and reduce the impact of stress on your body. Smoking and alcohol consumption are lifestyle choices that can significantly affect menopause. Smoking is linked to an earlier onset of menopause and can intensify symptoms like hot flashes. Alcohol can disrupt sleep patterns and worsen mood swings. Reducing or eliminating these habits can lead to a smoother menopausal transition.

Environmental factors also play a role in how menopause affects you. Exposure to endocrine-disrupting chemicals in many household products, plastics, and pesticides can interfere with your hormonal balance. These chemicals can mimic or block natural hormones, potentially worsening menopausal symptoms. Reducing exposure to these chemicals is advisable by choosing organic foods, using natural cleaning products, and avoiding plastic containers for food storage. Geographic location and climate can also influence the severity of symptoms. Some women in hotter climates experience more intense hot flashes, while some women in cooler regions find relief more easily.

You'll want to take a personalized approach to managing menopause. Each woman's experience is unique and influenced by genetic, lifestyle, and environmental factors. Personalizing your treatment and lifestyle changes based on your needs can make a significant difference. For instance, if you have a family history of osteoporosis, incorporating weight-bearing exercises and calcium-rich foods into your routine can help you maintain bone density. Similarly, if you are genetically predisposed to cardiovascular issues, focusing on heart-healthy habits like regular exercise and a balanced diet becomes even more critical.

Regular health checkups and monitoring are vital components of personalized menopause management. These checkups help identify any underlying health issues contributing to your symptoms. For example, thyroid dysfunction can mimic menopausal symptoms and should be ruled out or treated accordingly. Regular blood tests to monitor hormone levels, bone-density scans, and cardiovascular health assessments can provide a comprehensive picture of your health. Based on these test results, your healthcare provider can recommend appropriate treatments and lifestyle changes customized to your needs.

Remember, menopause is a natural phase of life that every woman experiences differently. There is no one-size-fits-all solution. Embracing a personalized approach that considers your unique genetic makeup, lifestyle habits, and environmental exposures can empower you to navigate menopause confidently. Regular checkups, a balanced diet, exercise, stress management, and reduced exposure to harmful chemicals can contribute to a smoother menopausal transition. Knowing you have the tools and knowledge to manage this phase can provide a sense of control and peace of mind. You are not alone in this journey; with the right strategies, you can thrive during and after menopause.

Chapter 2:

Managing Hot Flashes and

Night Sweats

Have you ever been in an important meeting, trying to focus on the discussion, when suddenly you felt a wave of heat rising from your chest to your face? Maybe your skin flushed, and beads of sweat formed on your forehead. You wanted to magically cool down, but you felt so self-conscious and uncomfortable. This is the reality of hot flashes, a common symptom of menopause that can strike at any moment. Managing these sudden bursts of heat and the accompanying night sweats is essential to maintaining your quality of life during menopause.

Immediate Relief Techniques for

Hot Flashes

A few immediate relief techniques can make a significant difference when a hot flash hits. One simple and effective method is using a handheld fan or portable cooling device; either one can provide instant relief by helping to lower your body temperature quickly. Keep a small fan in your purse or desk drawer so it's always within reach. Another quick cooling technique involves applying cold packs or cool cloths to the back of your neck. The neck area is particularly effective for cooling because it's rich in blood vessels. A cold compress can bring fast relief and help you feel more comfortable. You can also run cold water over your wrists for a similar effect.

Controlled Breathing

Controlled breathing exercises can also help mitigate the intensity of hot flashes. Deep breathing can calm your nervous system and reduce the severity of the hot flash. Start by finding a comfortable place to sit or stand. Close your eyes and take a slow, deep breath through your nose, allowing your abdomen to expand. Hold your breath for a few seconds, then exhale slowly through your mouth. Repeat this process several times until you feel the intensity of the hot flash subside. Another technique is paced respiration, which involves taking slow, deliberate breaths to help lower your body's stress response. Count to four as you inhale, hold for four counts, and then exhale for four counts. This rhythmic breathing can ease hot flash symptoms and help you regain your composure.

Staying hydrated is so important for managing hot flashes. Drinking cold water during a hot flash can help lower your body temperature from the inside out. Always keep a water bottle with you to take a sip whenever you feel a hot flash coming on. Staying hydrated also helps your body regulate its temperature more effectively, reducing the frequency and severity of hot flashes. Aim to drink at least eight glasses of water daily, and consider adding ice cubes to your drinks for an extra cooling effect.

The type of clothes you wear can also make a big difference when managing hot flashes. Layered, breathable clothing allows you to adjust to temperature changes easily. Choose moisture-wicking fabrics like cotton, bamboo, or moisture-wicking synthetics that can help keep you dry and comfortable.

Dressing in layers allows you to remove or add clothing to maintain a comfortable temperature. For example, you might start the day with a light cardigan over a sleeveless top, so you can quickly shed the cardigan if you feel a hot flash coming on. Loose-fitting clothes can also help improve air circulation around your body, reducing the likelihood of overheating.

Quick Cooling Checklist

- **Handheld fan:** Keep a small, portable fan with you for instant relief.

- **Cold packs:** Apply cold packs or cool cloths to your neck during a hot flash.

- **Hydration:** Drink cold water regularly and keep a water bottle handy.

- **Layered clothing:** Wear layers and choose moisture-wicking fabrics.

- **Deep breathing:** Practice deep-breathing exercises to calm your body.

Incorporating these immediate relief techniques into your daily routine can provide quick and effective ways to manage hot flashes. By staying prepared and knowing how to cool down quickly, you can reduce the discomfort and disruption caused by these sudden bursts of heat. Remember, you're not alone in this experience, and with the right strategies, you can navigate menopause with greater ease and confidence.

Diet and Hot Flashes: Foods to Include and to Avoid

You might be surprised to learn that what you eat can significantly impact the frequency and severity of your hot flashes. Certain foods contain compounds that help balance your hormones and reduce these uncomfortable episodes. Soy products, for instance, are rich in phytoestrogens. These plant-based compounds mimic estrogen in the body, providing a natural way to alleviate some menopausal symptoms. Including soy milk, tofu, and edamame in your diet can help stabilize your hormone levels and reduce hot flashes. Omega-3 fatty acids in fish like salmon and flaxseeds offer another support layer. These types of healthy fats have anti-inflammatory properties that help regulate your body's response to hormonal changes. Fruits and vegetables high in antioxidants, such as berries, spinach, and bell peppers, can also be beneficial. These foods help fight oxidative stress, which is linked to the severity of menopausal symptoms.

However, there are foods you should avoid, or at least cut back on, as well. Certain foods and beverages can trigger or worsen hot flashes. Caffeine and alcohol, for example, can expand blood vessels and increase body temperature, making hot flashes more likely. It's a good idea to limit your intake of coffee, tea, and alcoholic drinks. Spicy foods can also act as triggers. While some heat in your food might seem harmless, it can contribute to the sudden warmth you feel during a hot flash. Processed and sugary foods are another category to be cautious about. They can cause quick spikes and drops in blood sugar levels, which can destabilize your hormones and exacerbate hot flashes.

As stated previously, staying hydrated is another important aspect of managing hot flashes. Drinking plenty of water during the day helps regulate your body temperature and keeps your system running smoothly. Aim for at least eight glasses a day. Herbal teas such as chamomile or peppermint can also be soothing. Chamomile has calming properties that can help reduce stress levels, while peppermint offers a cooling sensation that can be particularly refreshing. Both options are caffeine-free, making them excellent choices for hydration without the risk of triggering hot flashes.

Incorporating hot flash–friendly foods into your daily meals doesn't have to be a hassle. Simple meal planning can make a big difference. Start your day with a breakfast that includes soy milk in your cereal or a smoothie. Consider a salad with leafy greens, cherry tomatoes, and grilled salmon for lunch. Add a sprinkle of flaxseeds for an extra boost of Omega-3s. Dinner can be a stir-fry with tofu, bell peppers, and broccoli, served over brown rice. Snacks are another opportunity to include beneficial foods. Fresh fruit, a handful of almonds, or sliced vegetables with hummus are all excellent choices that support your overall dietary goals.

Sample Meal Plan

- **Breakfast:** Soy milk smoothie with spinach, banana, and flaxseeds

- **Lunch:** Grilled salmon salad with mixed greens, cherry tomatoes, and a light vinaigrette

- **Dinner:** Tofu stir-fry with bell peppers, broccoli, and brown rice

- **Snacks:** Fresh fruit, almonds, and sliced vegetables with hummus

You can actively manage your hot flashes by making mindful choices about what you eat and drink. With the right foods, you can support your body and reduce the discomfort of hot flashes, making this phase of life more manageable.

Night Sweats: Creating a Sleep-Friendly Environment

Night sweats can disrupt your sleep, leaving you exhausted and irritable the next day. Creating a sleep-friendly environment can make a significant difference in managing night sweats. One of the first steps is optimizing your bedroom environment. Cooling mattress pads and pillows can help you regulate your body temperature throughout the night. These products are designed to dissipate heat and keep you cool, making it easier to stay asleep. Keeping the bedroom temperature cool with fans or air conditioning can also create a more comfortable sleeping environment. Aim for a room temperature between 60–67 °F, which is ideal for most people.

The type of bedding and sleepwear you choose also plays an important role in managing night sweats. Opt for light, breathable fabrics like cotton or bamboo—they are excellent at wicking moisture away from your skin, keeping you dry and comfortable. Avoid heavy blankets and opt for layers instead. Layering allows you to adjust your bedding to suit your comfort level throughout the night. Moisture-wicking sheets and pajamas are particularly effective. These products are designed to draw sweat away from your body, helping you stay cool and dry. Investing in high-quality, breathable bedding can significantly improve your sleep quality.

Establishing a pre-sleep routine can also help minimize night sweats. A cool shower or bath before bed lowers your body temperature, making it easier to fall asleep. The cooling effect of water can be incredibly soothing, helping you relax before bedtime. Avoiding heavy meals and spicy foods close to bedtime is another important step, as these can increase your body temperature and trigger night sweats. Instead, try a light snack if you're hungry before bed. Yogurt or a small handful of nuts can be satisfying without causing you any discomfort.

You'll need to incorporate good sleep hygiene practices into your routine to improve the quality of your sleep. Maintaining a regular sleep schedule can regulate your body's internal clock, which helps you fall asleep and wake up at the same time each day. Phones, tablets, and computers emit blue light that can interfere with your body's production of melatonin, a hormone that regulates sleep. Instead of scrolling through your phone before bed, read a book or practice gentle stretching exercises.

Practicing relaxation techniques before bed can further improve your sleep quality. Techniques such as deep-breathing exercises, muscle relaxation, and meditation can help calm your mind and prepare your body for sleep. Reading a book or listening to soothing music can also help you wind down before bed. Creating a bedtime routine that includes these relaxation techniques can signal to your body that it's time to sleep, making it easier to fall asleep and stay asleep.

Creating a Sleep-Friendly Environment Checklist

- **Cooling mattress pads and pillows:** Invest in products that regulate body temperature.

- **Room temperature:** Keep the bedroom cool with fans or air conditioning (60–67 °F).

- **Breathable bedding:** Choose light, moisture-wicking fabrics like cotton or bamboo.

- **Layering:** Use layers instead of heavy blankets to adjust comfort levels.

- **Pre-sleep cool shower:** Take a cool shower or bath before bed.

- **Avoid heavy meals:** Skip heavy and/or spicy foods close to bedtime.

- **Regular sleep schedule:** Stick to a consistent sleep and wake-up time.

- **Limit screen time:** Avoid screens starting at least an hour before bed.

- **Relaxation techniques:** Practice deep breathing, meditation, or gentle stretching.

You can significantly reduce the impact of night sweats by adjusting your sleep environment and routine. A cool, comfortable bedroom, good sleep hygiene, and relaxation techniques can help you achieve a more restful and rejuvenating night's sleep. Managing night sweats effectively can improve your overall quality of life, allowing you to face each day with more energy and a positive outlook.

Prescriptions and Supplements for Hot Flashes and Night Sweats

When hot flashes and night sweats become overwhelming, prescription medications can offer significant relief. One of the most well-known options is hormone replacement therapy (HRT). HRT involves the use of estrogen, either alone or combined with progesterone, to help manage menopausal symptoms. For women who have had a hysterectomy, estrogen-only therapy is usually recommended. For those who still have their uterus, combined estrogen-progesterone therapy is used. The benefits of HRT include a significant reduction in the frequency and intensity of hot flashes and night sweats and improvements in sleep quality and overall mood. However, you need to be aware of the potential risks associated with HRT, such as an increased risk of breast cancer, blood clots, and stroke. Therefore, a personalized approach to HRT, tailored to your individual health profile and needs, is important. Your healthcare provider will help you determine the most effective dose and the appropriate duration of treatment to minimize risks.

Nonhormonal Medications

For those who cannot or choose not to use HRT, nonhormonal medications offer alternative treatment options. Antidepressants, such as selective serotonin reuptake inhibitors (SSRIs) and serotonin-norepinephrine reuptake inhibitors (SNRIs), have been found to reduce hot flashes. These medications can help manage symptoms without using hormones and work by altering the brain's chemical pathways that regulate mood and body temperature. Alternatively, some anti-seizure medications can also reduce the frequency and intensity of hot flashes. While nonhormonal medicines can be effective, they also come with potential side effects, such as dizziness, dry mouth, and fatigue. It's important to discuss these options with your healthcare provider to determine the best course of action for your situation.

Herbal Supplements

Herbal supplements are another avenue that many women explore for managing menopausal symptoms. Black cohosh is one of the most commonly used herbal remedies for hot flashes and night sweats. It is believed to have estrogen-like effects on the body, which can help balance hormones and alleviate symptoms. Red clover, another herbal supplement, contains isoflavones that mimic estrogen and can provide some relief. However, the safety and efficacy of herbal supplements can vary, and the FDA does not regulate them as they do with prescription medications, so before starting any herbal supplement, consult your healthcare provider to ensure it is safe and appropriate for you. Some supplements can interact with medications you may already be taking, so professional guidance is important.

Consulting healthcare providers for personalized treatment plans is vital when managing menopause symptoms. Understanding the variety of professionals in the field can be confusing. Options include consulting medical doctors (MDs), who practice conventional medicine and can prescribe a range of medications; doctors of osteopathic medicine (DOs), who have a holistic approach but can also prescribe medication; and naturopathic doctors (NDs), who focus on natural remedies and holistic treatments. Understanding each one's unique qualifications and methods can help you decide which type of provider aligns best with your treatment preferences. Before your appointment, prepare a detailed list of your symptoms, including their frequency and impact, so you are prepared to have a comprehensive discussion with your healthcare provider. Sharing your treatment preferences and openness to medical or natural interventions will enable your provider to create a plan that suits your needs. Ongoing communication for monitoring and adjusting your treatment plan is key to ensuring its effectiveness and your safety.

In this chapter, we've explored various options for managing hot flashes and night sweats. From HRT to nonhormonal medications and herbal supplements, there are multiple options to consider. Consulting healthcare providers for personalized treatment plans is crucial for finding the right solution for you. As we move forward, we'll explore the many ways in which menopause affects your sleep habits, how to sleep better, and strategies for living a better-rested life.

Chapter 3:

Sleep Disturbances

and Insomnia

Menopausal insomnia disrupts the lives of countless women. If you suffer from this, you might find yourself lying in bed awake after midnight, glancing at your clock to see that somehow, another hour has slipped by, yet sleep remains elusive. You toss and turn, your mind racing, and when you finally drift off, it feels like mere seconds before you're jolted awake again. This cycle repeats night after night, leaving you exhausted and frustrated.

Understanding Menopausal Insomnia

Menopausal insomnia is a common and often debilitating symptom of menopause and is characterized by various sleep disturbances that can severely impact your quality of life. One of the most prevalent issues is difficulty falling asleep. You may lie awake for hours, unable to quiet your mind or relax your body enough to drift off. Frequent waking during the night is another hallmark of menopausal insomnia. You might wake up multiple times, sometimes every hour, making achieving deep, restorative sleep impossible. Early-morning awakenings, when you wake up much earlier than intended and cannot fall back asleep, are also common. Even if you manage to sleep for a few hours, the sleep you get often feels nonrestorative. You wake up feeling just as tired as when you went to bed, if not more so.

The causes of menopausal insomnia are multifaceted and often interrelated. Hormonal fluctuations play a significant role. The decline in estrogen and progesterone affects your body's ability to regulate sleep. Estrogen, for instance, influences the production of serotonin, a neurotransmitter that helps regulate sleep. Lower estrogen levels can disrupt this balance, making falling and staying asleep harder. Progesterone, known for its calming and sedative effects, also decreases during menopause, contributing to sleep difficulties. Hot flashes and night sweats can further exacerbate insomnia, waking you up multiple times a night and leaving you feeling restless and uncomfortable. Anxiety and depression are also common during menopause and can significantly impact your sleep. It's hard to achieve restful sleep when worries about aging, health, and changes in your life keep you up at night.

Insomnia not only affects your nights, it also takes a toll on your daily life. Chronic fatigue and daytime sleepiness are often the first noticeable impacts. Insomnia can make it challenging to get through the day without feeling exhausted. This relentless fatigue can affect your ability to concentrate, remember things, and complete daily tasks efficiently. Impaired cognitive function becomes a significant issue, with memory lapses and difficulty focusing becoming more frequent. These cognitive struggles can affect your work performance and personal life, increasing stress and frustration. Mood disturbances are another common consequence of insomnia and can make you more irritable, anxious, and prone to mood swings, straining your relationships with family, friends, and colleagues, further adding to your stress.

The long-term health risks associated with untreated insomnia are substantial. Chronic sleep deprivation increases your risk of cardiovascular diseases. Studies have shown that poor sleep can lead to hypertension, heart disease, and even stroke. Sleep loss can also weaken your immune system, causing other significant risks. Sleep is necessary for immune function, and consistently missing out on restorative sleep can make you more susceptible to infections and illnesses. Anxiety and depression can be consequences of sleep disturbances, creating a vicious cycle that is difficult to break. Addressing insomnia effectively and seeking appropriate treatment can reduce these risks.

Insomnia Self-Assessment Checklist

- Difficulty falling asleep

- Frequent waking during the night

- Early-morning awakenings

- Feeling tired despite sleeping

- Daytime fatigue and sleepiness

- Memory lapses and difficulty concentrating

- Mood swings and irritability

Understanding menopausal insomnia and its wide-reaching effects is the first step in managing it. By recognizing the symptoms and their causes, you can begin to take proactive measures to improve your sleep and overall well-being.

Sleep Apnea

Sleep apnea is a disorder in which your breathing repeatedly stops and starts during sleep. This can lead to severe disruptions in your rest, and it's more common than you might think, especially among women going through menopause. Obstructive sleep apnea (OSA) is the most common type. During OSA, the muscles in your throat relax too much, blocking your airway. Symptoms of sleep apnea typically include:

- Snoring

- Gasping for air during sleep

- Waking up with a dry mouth

- Morning headaches

- Feeling excessively sleepy during the day

You might also experience difficulty concentrating as well as mood changes.

Weight gain during menopause can increase the risk of developing sleep apnea. As your metabolism slows and hormonal changes prompt your body to store more fat, particularly around the neck and upper airway, this added weight can obstruct your breathing. If you find yourself gaining weight, it's worth monitoring your sleep quality and looking for any signs of sleep apnea. Hormonal fluctuations can also contribute to changes in muscle tone around your airway, making it more likely to collapse during sleep.

The risks associated with sleep apnea are significant and can affect various aspects of your health. One primary concern is the increased risk of cardiovascular diseases. Interrupted breathing during sleep leads to drops in blood oxygen levels, which puts a strain on your heart and can raise your blood pressure, increasing the likelihood of heart disease and stroke. High blood pressure itself can become a chronic condition if sleep apnea goes untreated. Sleep apnea is also linked to insulin resistance, which raises your risk of developing type 2 diabetes. The constant cycle of waking and sleeping disrupts the restorative processes of the brain, leading to changes in mood and cognitive function. You might find yourself more irritable, anxious, or depressed. The lack of restful sleep impairs memory and concentration, making daily tasks more challenging. This increases your risk of accidents at home and on the road. All these compounded health risks can shorten your lifespan.

If you suspect you have sleep apnea, you need to seek medical advice. Diagnostic sleep studies are the gold standard for identifying sleep apnea. Depending on your healthcare provider's recommendation, these studies can be conducted in a sleep lab or at home. During a sleep study, you'll be monitored for various physiological signals, including your breathing patterns, oxygen levels, heart rate, and brain activity. This comprehensive monitoring helps diagnose the severity of your sleep apnea and determine the best course of treatment.

Therapeutic sleep studies might follow the initial diagnosis to fine-tune your treatment. One of the most effective treatments for sleep apnea is the use of continuous positive airway pressure (CPAP). A CPAP device delivers a constant stream of air through a mask, keeping your airway open and preventing interruptions in your breathing. Adherence to CPAP therapy can significantly improve your sleep quality, reduce daytime sleepiness, and lower your risk of associated health issues. Other treatment options include lifestyle changes such as weight loss, exercise, positional therapy to prevent back-sleeping, and, in some cases, surgery.

Understanding sleep apnea and its implications is the first step toward managing this condition. Proper diagnosis and treatment can dramatically improve your quality of life and overall health. If you experience sleep apnea symptoms, consider discussing them with your healthcare provider to explore the best diagnostic and treatment options for you.

Natural Remedies for Better Sleep

When it comes to improving sleep during menopause, natural remedies can be pretty effective. Melatonin is one such remedy. This hormone plays a crucial role in regulating your sleep-wake cycle. Your body naturally produces melatonin in response to darkness, signaling it's time to sleep. However, melatonin levels can decline as you age, making it harder to fall asleep. Taking melatonin supplements can help realign your sleep patterns. It's best to start with a low dose of around 0.5–1 milligram, taken 30 minutes to an hour before bedtime. You can gradually increase the dosage, if needed, but it's always wise to consult your healthcare provider first.

Magnesium is another mineral that can significantly improve sleep quality. It helps relax muscles and reduce stress, making falling and staying asleep easier. Magnesium supports the production of GABA, a neurotransmitter that promotes relaxation and sleep. You can find magnesium in supplements and various foods like leafy greens, nuts, seeds, and whole grains. A warm bath with Epsom salts, rich in magnesium, can also be a soothing pre-sleep ritual. Taking a magnesium supplement of around 200–400 milligrams per day can be beneficial, but again, consult your healthcare provider to ensure it's right for you.

Herbal supplements have long been used to aid sleep; several are particularly effective for menopausal women. Valerian root is known for its calming effects. It has been used for centuries to treat insomnia and anxiety. Taking valerian root about an hour before bed can increase relaxation and help you drift off more easily. Chamomile is another excellent option. A cup of chamomile tea before bed can be very soothing, helping to reduce anxiety and promote sleep. Lemon balm and passionflower are also worth considering. Lemon balm is high in antioxidants and can improve sleep quality, especially when combined with valerian. Passionflower is often used as a sedative and can help with sleep, mood, and hot flashes.

Always consult a healthcare provider before starting any new supplement. Certain supplements can interact with medications you may already be taking, leading to unwanted side effects. You need to monitor your body's response to any new supplement and adjust the dosage as needed. If you have sleep apnea, be cautious with sleep supplements, as they can sometimes worsen your condition. Your healthcare provider can guide you in choosing the right supplements and dosages for your specific needs.

Essential oils and aromatherapy can create a calming bedtime routine that promotes sleep. Lavender oil is particularly well-known for its relaxing properties. You can use a few drops in a diffuser to fill your bedroom with a soothing scent. Roman chamomile oil is another great option. Its calming effect can help prepare your mind and body for sleep. You can also use these oils in a pillow spray or add a few drops to your bath for extra relaxation.

Relaxation Techniques

Relaxation techniques are another powerful tool for improving sleep quality. Progressive muscle relaxation involves creating tension and then slowly releasing each muscle, starting from your toes and working up to your head. This technique helps release stress and prepare your body for sleep. Guided imagery is another effective method that can distract your mind from daily stresses and create a sense of calm. Close your eyes and imagine a peaceful scene. Focus on the details, like the sound of the waves or the rustling of leaves. Deep-breathing exercises are also very effective. You can help lower your heart rate and promote relaxation by inhaling slowly through your nose for four seconds, holding your breath for seven seconds, and then exhaling slowly through your mouth for eight seconds.

Another practice that can reduce stress and anxiety, making it easier to fall asleep and significantly improve sleep quality, is mindfulness meditation. This type of meditation involves focusing on the present moment by being aware of your surroundings and can be as simple as concentrating on touch, sound, sight, smell, or taste. Body-scan meditation is another helpful technique. Start at your toes and move up to your head, noticing any sensations or tension. Many apps and resources are available that offer guided meditation sessions to help you sleep. These can be a valuable addition to your nighttime routine, helping you achieve more restful and rejuvenating sleep.

Sleep Hygiene: Creating a Restful Environment

Creating an optimal sleep environment to improve sleep quality during menopause is important. Keeping the bedroom cool and dark can make a significant difference. During sleep, your body temperature naturally drops, so maintaining a cooler room between 60–67 °F can help with this process. Using blackout curtains can also be beneficial. Blackout curtains block out any external light while creating a dark environment that signals to your brain it's time to sleep. If blackout curtains aren't an option, consider using an eye mask. This simple accessory can effectively block out light, making falling and staying asleep easier. Noise can be another barrier to restful sleep. White noise machines or earplugs can minimize noise and help create a peaceful environment. Earplugs block out disruptive sounds, while white noise machines can mask background noise, providing a consistent and soothing soundscape.

Establishing a consistent bedtime routine is another fundamental aspect of good sleep hygiene, which reinforces your sleep-wake cycle, making it easier to fall asleep and wake up naturally. Limiting stimulating activities before bed is also essential. Activities like watching TV, browsing on your phone, or engaging in intense conversations can make it harder for your mind to wind down. Instead, incorporate calming activities into your bedtime routine. Reading a book, listening to soothing music, or practicing gentle stretching exercises can signal to your body that it's time to relax. These activities can create a sense of calm and make the transition to sleep smoother.

Limiting Screen Time

Screen time can significantly impact your sleep quality—blue light emitted by phones, tablets, and computers can interfere with your body's production of melatonin, a hormone that regulates sleep. To mitigate this, avoid screens at least an hour before bed. If you must use your devices, consider using blue-light filters or apps designed to reduce blue-light exposure. These filters can help minimize the impact on your sleep. Setting boundaries with your screen time can make a noticeable difference in how easily you fall asleep and the quality of your rest.

Limiting Nighttime Caffeine and Meals

Your diet also plays a significant role in sleep quality. Avoiding caffeine and heavy meals close to bedtime can prevent disruptions in your sleep. Caffeine can stay in your system for several hours, making it harder to fall asleep. Try to avoid caffeinated beverages like coffee, tea, and soda in the afternoon and evening. Heavy meals can cause discomfort and indigestion, which can keep you awake. Instead, opt for a light, sleep-friendly snack if you feel hungry before bed. A banana or a small handful of nuts can provide the necessary nutrients without causing discomfort. These snacks contain tryptophan and magnesium, which can help promote relaxation and better sleep.

Incorporating these practices into your daily routine can create a more restful environment, making it easier to achieve quality sleep. By optimizing your sleep environment, establishing a consistent bedtime routine, managing screen time, and making mindful dietary choices, you can set the stage for better sleep and improved overall well-being. Remember, small changes can significantly improve your sleep quality and quality of life.

Cognitive Behavioral Therapy for Insomnia (CBT-I)

Cognitive behavioral therapy for Insomnia (CBT-I) is a highly effective treatment for sleep disturbances, particularly those experienced during menopause. Unlike medication, which often provides only temporary relief, CBT-I offers long-term solutions by addressing the underlying issues that disrupt sleep. This therapy works by changing the thoughts and behaviors that contribute to insomnia. Through a series of structured sessions, CBT-I helps you develop healthier sleep habits and alter negative thought patterns that make sleep difficult. One key benefit of CBT-I compared to medication is its durability. While sleep medications can lose their effectiveness over time and have side effects, CBT-I equips you with skills that can help you manage insomnia for the rest of your life.

Cognitive techniques in CBT-I focus on identifying and challenging negative sleep thoughts. Many people struggling with insomnia develop a fear of not being able to sleep, which only worsens the problem. By recognizing these irrational thoughts, you can challenge and reframe them. For instance, if you constantly worry about not getting enough sleep and how it will affect your next day, CBT-I teaches you to reframe this thinking. Instead of catastrophizing, you might tell yourself, *Even if I don't sleep well, I can still function and get through the day.* Reframing catastrophic thinking into more balanced, realistic thoughts can reduce anxiety around sleep, making it easier to relax and drift off.

Behavioral Techniques

Behavioral techniques are another cornerstone of CBT-I. Sleep-restriction therapy is one such technique that can be remarkably effective. This method involves limiting your time in bed to the actual amount of time you sleep. If you typically spend eight hours in bed but only sleep for five, you would initially restrict your time in bed to five hours. This process can help build a stronger association between bed and sleep, making it easier to fall and stay asleep. Another behavioral technique is stimulus control therapy, which aims to break the association between the bed and activities that aren't conducive to sleep, like watching TV or worrying. By only using your bed for sleep and sex, you can strengthen the mental connection that bed means sleep. Relaxation training, including progressive muscle relaxation and deep-breathing exercises, can also help reduce physical tension and mental stress, making it easier to fall asleep.

Implementing CBT-I techniques at home can be straightforward and empowering. Keeping a sleep diary is a crucial first step. Track your sleep patterns, noting when you go to bed, how long it takes you to fall asleep, how often you wake up, and how you feel in the morning. This information can help you identify patterns and triggers that affect your sleep. Setting realistic sleep goals is another important aspect. Instead of aiming for a perfect night's sleep immediately, set small, achievable goals like reducing the time it takes to fall asleep by 15 minutes. If you find it challenging to implement these techniques on your own, seeking professional help can be beneficial. A trained CBT-I therapist can guide you through the process, offering personalized strategies and support.

Incorporating CBT-I into your routine can significantly improve your sleep quality and overall well-being. The skills you learn are not just for managing insomnia but also helping you handle other stressors in life. As you navigate menopause, these techniques can provide a stable foundation for better sleep and mental health. Combining cognitive and behavioral strategies can offer lasting relief from insomnia. Now, as we move forward, we will explore the emotional and mental well-being aspects of menopause, providing you with methods to maintain balance and strength during this significant life transition.

Chapter 4:

Emotional and Mental

Well-Being

Menopause is an unpredictable emotional rollercoaster, a ride that many women have suffered through. You could be sitting at dinner, laughing with your family, when a wave of irritability washes over you. You snap at your loved ones unexpectedly, leaving you feeling guilty and confused because you didn't see the wave coming. Hormonal fluctuations can wreak havoc on your mood, causing anxiety and irritability. Understanding the root causes of these mood swings is the first step in managing them effectively.

Coping With Mood Swings and Anxiety

During menopause, your body undergoes significant hormonal changes—mainly estrogen and progesterone, which play a pivotal role in regulating your mood. Estrogen, for instance, interacts with neurotransmitters such as serotonin, often called the "feel-good" chemical. When estrogen levels fluctuate, it can disrupt serotonin production, leading to mood swings, anxiety, and even depression. Progesterone, known for its calming effects, also declines during menopause, further contributing to emotional instability. These hormonal shifts can make you feel like you're on an emotional seesaw, with highs and lows that can be challenging to manage.

Daily coping strategies can make a significant difference in managing mood swings. Keeping a mood journal is a practical tool that can help you track patterns and triggers. By noting your emotional highs and lows, you can identify what exacerbates your mood swings and take steps to mitigate those triggers. Regular physical activity is another effective strategy. Engaging in exercises like walking, swimming, or yoga releases endorphins, which are the body's natural mood lifters. Physical activity also helps regulate your sleep patterns, further stabilizing your mood.

Natural remedies and supplements offer additional avenues for managing mood swings. Omega-3 fatty acids, found in fish oil and flaxseeds, have been shown to improve moods and reduce symptoms of depression. These healthy fats support brain function and can help balance your emotional state. St. John's Wort is another herbal remedy known for its mood-stabilizing properties. However, it's essential to consult a healthcare provider before starting any new supplement, as St. John's Wort can interact with other medications. Safety considerations should be a top priority, especially if you already take prescribed medication for other health conditions.

You should seek professional help when mood swings and anxiety become overwhelming. Consulting a mental health professional can provide the support and tools to manage your symptoms effectively. Cognitive Behavioral Therapy (CBT) is a well-established treatment that may help you reframe negative thought patterns and develop healthier coping mechanisms. For severe mood swings, medication options are available. Antidepressants, such as selective serotonin reuptake inhibitors (SSRIs), can help balance the chemicals in your brain and improve your mood. These medications are often prescribed along with therapy to provide a comprehensive treatment plan.

Mood Journal Prompt

- **Morning:** How do you feel when you wake up? (e.g., anxious, calm, or neutral)

- **Afternoon:** Note any significant mood changes. What were you doing? (e.g., work or socializing)

- **Evening:** Reflect on your mood before bed. Did any specific events or interactions affect it?

- **Triggers:** Identify any patterns or common triggers (e.g., stress at work or dietary choices).

- **Coping strategies:** What helped you manage your mood today? (e.g., exercise or talking to a friend)

Dealing With Brain Fog and Memory Issues

Have you ever walked into a room and completely forgotten why you went there in the first place? Or maybe you find yourself repeatedly asking the same question because you can't recall the answer. These moments of forgetfulness and difficulty concentrating are often referred to as "brain fog," a common symptom of menopause that can make everyday tasks feel like monumental challenges. Brain fog can manifest as difficulty retaining information, trouble focusing on tasks, and a general sense of mental cloudiness. It's as if a thick fog has settled over your mind, obscuring your usual clarity and sharpness.

The causes of brain fog during menopause are multifaceted but largely stem from hormonal changes. As estrogen levels fluctuate and decline, this hormone's influence on cognitive functions becomes evident. Estrogen helps regulate neurotransmitters in the brain, including acetylcholine, which is vital for memory and learning. When estrogen levels drop, the production and regulation of these neurotransmitters can be disrupted, leading to cognitive difficulties. Additionally, the stress and anxiety that often accompany menopause can further exacerbate brain fog, creating a vicious cycle that makes it challenging to break free from this mental haze.

How to Lift the Fog

Combating brain fog involves a combination of lifestyle changes and targeted strategies to support brain health. Exercise is one of the most effective ways to improve circulation and blood flow to the brain. Physical activity increases oxygen delivery to brain cells, promoting overall cognitive function. Try to do at least 30 minutes of moderate exercise on most days of the week. Activities like brisk walking, swimming, or even dancing can make a significant difference. Regular exercise also helps reduce stress, a known contributor to brain fog.

Get Enough Sleep

Getting enough sleep is pivotal for cognitive health. During sleep, your brain consolidates memories and removes toxins that can impair function. Aim for 7–9 hours of quality sleep each night. Establishing a regular sleep routine, avoiding caffeine and electronics before bed, and creating a restful sleep environment can help improve the quality of your rest. Stay hydrated, as dehydration can lead to memory and concentration issues. Drinking water throughout the day ensures your brain stays well-hydrated and functions optimally.

Eat a Healthy Diet

Eating a healthy diet low in fat and rich in nutrients supports brain health. Focus on consuming foods high in antioxidants, such as berries, leafy greens, and nuts. These foods help combat oxidative stress, which can damage brain cells. Omega-3 fatty acids, found in fatty fish like salmon and flaxseeds, are particularly beneficial for cognitive function. They support the structure of brain cells and help reduce inflammation. Avoiding processed foods and excessive sugar can also help maintain your mental clarity.

Try Hormone Therapy

Hormone therapy can be another effective way to address brain fog. By supplementing estrogen, hormone therapy can help stabilize the hormonal fluctuations that contribute to cognitive difficulties. This can lead to improved memory, concentration, and overall cognitive function. However, hormone therapy is not suitable for everyone and comes with its own set of risks and benefits. You'll need to consult a healthcare provider to determine whether hormone therapy is the right option for you.

By incorporating regular exercise, ensuring adequate sleep, staying well-hydrated, and eating a nutrient-rich diet, you can significantly reduce the impact of brain fog. Additionally, exploring hormone therapy with your healthcare provider may offer further relief. These steps can help you regain mental clarity and navigate menopause with confidence.

Mindfulness and Meditation Techniques

Mindfulness is the practice of paying attention to the present moment. If you are mindful, you are aware of your thoughts, feelings, and sensations as they occur. For many women, menopause brings a whirlwind of emotions and physical changes that can be overwhelming. Practicing mindfulness can help reduce stress and anxiety, offering a sense of calm amid the storm. By focusing on the present, you can better regulate your emotions and respond to challenges with greater clarity and composure. This practice helps you create a mental space where you can observe your experiences without being swept away by them, making it easier to cope with the ups and downs of menopause.

Breathing Exercises

One of the simplest ways to incorporate mindfulness into your daily life is through breathing exercises. Start by finding a quiet space where you won't be disturbed. Sit comfortably and close your eyes. Take a deep breath through your nose, allowing your belly to expand. Hold your breath for a moment, then exhale slowly through your mouth. Focus on the sensation of the breath entering and leaving your body. If your mind wanders, gently bring your attention back to your breathing. Practicing this exercise for a few minutes daily can help you feel more centered and relaxed. Another effective technique is the body scan meditation. Lie down in a comfortable position and close your eyes. Starting from your toes, slowly bring awareness to each part of your body, noticing any sensations, tension, or discomfort. Move your attention up through your legs, torso, arms, and head, taking time with each body part. This practice can help you reconnect with your body and release any tension you might be holding.

Mindful Walking

Mindful walking is another accessible practice that can be easily integrated into your daily routine. Find a quiet place where you can walk without distractions, such as a park or a quiet street. Begin walking slowly and deliberately, paying close attention to the sensation of your feet touching the ground. Notice the movement of your legs and the rhythm of your breath. If your mind starts to wander, gently bring your focus back to the act of walking. This practice can help you develop a sense of presence and mindfulness even during everyday activities.

Guided Meditation

Guided meditation sessions can be incredibly helpful for those new to mindfulness or seeking additional guidance. Popular meditation apps, such as Headspace, Calm, Smiling Mind, and more, offer a wide range of guided meditations that cater to different needs and preferences. These apps provide structured sessions to help you develop a consistent mindfulness practice. Online platforms also offer free guided meditations, allowing you to explore different techniques and find what works best. You can find sessions focused on relaxation, stress reduction, and emotional balance, making it easier to address specific challenges you may face during menopause.

Incorporating mindfulness into your daily life doesn't have to be complicated. Mindful eating is a simple yet powerful practice that can transform your relationship with food. Start by paying attention to the colors, textures, and smells of your meal. Take small bites and chew slowly, savoring each mouthful. Notice the sensations in your body while you eat, such as the feeling of fullness or satisfaction. This practice can help you develop a more mindful and balanced approach to eating, reducing overeating and promoting better digestion. Mindfulness can also be practiced while performing chores or commuting. For example, while washing dishes, pay attention to the sensation of the water on your hands and the sound of the dishes clinking. During your commute, observe your surroundings and notice the sights and sounds without judgment. Setting aside time for a daily mindfulness routine, even if it's just a few minutes, can help you create a sense of presence and calm throughout your day.

Cognitive Behavioral Therapy (CBT) for Emotional Health

Cognitive behavioral therapy, as discussed in Chapter 3 and often called CBT, is a form of psychotherapy that focuses on changing negative thought patterns and behaviors. For women going through menopause, CBT offers a structured way to manage emotional challenges such as anxiety and depression. At its core, CBT works by identifying and challenging distorted thinking patterns that contribute to emotional distress. By reframing these thoughts, you can alter the emotional and behavioral responses that follow. This form of therapy is particularly relevant during menopause when hormonal fluctuations can exacerbate feelings of anxiety and depression.

One of the most powerful aspects of CBT is its ability to bring about lasting change. By working to change thought patterns, CBT helps you understand the connection between your thoughts, emotions, and actions. For example, if you often think, *I'm never going to feel better*, this negative thought can lead to feelings of hopelessness and inactivity. CBT helps you challenge this thought by examining the evidence for and against it, ultimately leading to a more balanced perspective. This shift in thinking can reduce anxiety and depression, providing you with tools to manage these emotions more effectively.

Specific CBT techniques can be beneficial for reducing anxiety. One such technique is identifying and challenging anxious thoughts. Start by recognizing the thoughts that trigger your anxiety. For instance, you might think, *What if I can't handle my responsibilities?* Once identified, challenge these thoughts by asking yourself if they are based on facts or assumptions. Often, you'll find that these thoughts are exaggerated or unfounded. Another effective technique is exposure therapy, which involves gradually facing the situations that trigger your anxiety. In a controlled and supportive environment, you can desensitize yourself to these triggers, reducing their power over you.

When it comes to managing depression, CBT offers several effective strategies. Behavioral activation, which focuses on counteracting inactivity, is one such technique. Depression often leads to withdrawal from activities that once brought joy. Behavioral activation encourages you to schedule and engage in these activities, even when you don't feel like it. This can help break the cycle of inactivity and low mood. Cognitive restructuring is another valuable strategy. This involves identifying negative thought patterns and replacing them with more balanced and realistic ones. For example, instead of thinking, *I'm a failure*, you might reframe it to, *I've faced challenges, but I've also had successes.*

You need to contact a professional for support if you are feeling severely anxious or depressed. While self-help techniques can be beneficial, consulting a mental health professional can provide customized strategies and support. A therapist trained in CBT can guide you through these techniques, helping you apply them effectively to your situation. In some cases, medication may be necessary to manage severe symptoms. Antidepressants, such as SSRIs, can help balance brain chemicals and improve your mood. These medications are often most effective when used with therapy.

The structured approach of CBT makes it a powerful tool for managing the emotional challenges of menopause. Changing negative thought patterns and engaging in positive behaviors can significantly improve your emotional well-being. Whether you work with a therapist or explore CBT techniques alone, the skills you learn can help you through this phase of life with more confidence and self-reflection.

Building a Support Network

Managing menopause can be a lonely and isolating experience, but having a strong support network can make a world of difference. The emotional and psychological benefits of social support are immense. When you have people to lean on, your burden feels lighter. Sharing your experiences, fears, and triumphs with others who understand can reduce feelings of isolation. Social support provides a sense of belonging and validation, reminding you that you are not alone. Having a support network can also improve your mental health by reducing stress and anxiety, helping you create a more positive outlook on life.

Finding support groups, both local and online, is a great way to connect with others who are going through similar experiences. Local menopause support groups can offer face-to-face interaction, allowing you to build relationships with women in your community. These groups often meet regularly, providing a safe space to share stories, ask questions, and offer support. If you prefer the convenience and anonymity of online interactions, numerous communities and forums focus on menopause. Social media groups and specialized health forums host vibrant, supportive communities where you can find advice, share experiences, and form connections. The benefits of shared experiences and peer support in these groups are invaluable. Knowing that others have faced and overcome the same challenges can provide hope and practical solutions.

Open communication with family and friends is necessary for building a supportive home environment. Talking about menopause with your partner and children can help them understand what you're going through. Explain the symptoms you experience and how they affect your daily life, making it easier for them to offer the support you need. Educating your loved ones about menopausal symptoms can also dispel myths and reduce misunderstandings. A supportive home environment can significantly impact your emotional well-being, providing a sanctuary where you feel understood and cared for.

Professional support networks are another vital component of managing menopause. Consulting healthcare providers for comprehensive care ensures that you receive the medical support you need. Your doctor can help you explore treatment options, manage symptoms, and monitor your overall health. Mental health professionals can provide emotional support, helping you cope with the psychological challenges of menopause. Therapy can offer strategies for managing stress, anxiety, and depression, improving your quality of life. Holistic practitioners, such as nutritionists, acupuncturists, and herbalists, can offer integrated care that addresses your physical, emotional, and spiritual well-being. Combining conventional and holistic approaches can provide a balanced, comprehensive support system.

Building a strong support network can significantly impact your menopause experience. Emotional and social support from peers, family, and professionals can provide the understanding and care you need. As we move forward, we will explore the physical aspects of menopause, focusing on managing weight and maintaining a healthy metabolism.

Chapter 5:

Weight Management and

Metabolism

Many menopausal women have been in this situation: You're standing in front of your closet, frustrated because nothing fits right anymore. You've been diligent about your diet and exercise, yet the weight seems to cling stubbornly, particularly around your abdomen. The changes in your body can feel disheartening, but understanding the metabolic shifts at play can empower you to manage your weight more effectively.

Understanding Metabolic Changes in Menopause

During menopause, hormonal changes significantly impact your metabolism. The decline in estrogen levels plays a central role in this process. Estrogen helps regulate body fat distribution, and its reduction leads to increased fat accumulation, particularly around the abdomen. This shift from a more even fat distribution to a centralized one can be physically and emotionally challenging. Clothes fit differently, and the weight around your middle is harder to lose. This isn't just a cosmetic issue; abdominal fat is closely linked to various health risks.

Decreased muscle mass is another critical factor contributing to a slower metabolism during menopause. Muscle tissue burns more calories than fat tissue, even at rest. As muscle mass declines, your body's basal metabolic rate (BMR) also decreases, meaning you burn fewer calories throughout the day, which can lead to weight gain, even if your diet and physical activity levels remain unchanged. Maintaining and building muscle through resistance training can help counteract this decline and support a more stable metabolism.

Insulin resistance is another metabolic challenge that often accompanies menopause. Insulin is a hormone that helps regulate blood sugar levels. During menopause, your body can become less responsive to insulin, leading to higher blood sugar levels and increased fat storage. This condition makes weight management more difficult and raises your risk of developing type 2 diabetes. Recognizing the signs of insulin resistance, such as increased cravings for sugary foods and unexplained weight gain, is vital for early intervention and management.

Common Symptoms of Metabolic Changes

The common symptoms and signs of these metabolic changes can be subtle but significant. Increased abdominal fat is often one of the first noticeable changes. You might find that your waistline expands, even if your overall weight remains stable. Slower energy expenditure is another symptom. You may feel more tired than usual, and activities that once energized you might now leave you feeling drained. Changes in appetite and cravings can also signal metabolic shifts. You might crave more high-sugar or high-fat foods, further complicating weight management.

The long-term health risks associated with unmanaged metabolic changes during menopause are substantial. One of the most significant risks is the higher likelihood of developing type 2 diabetes. Insulin resistance, if left unchecked, can progress to diabetes, a condition that requires lifelong management. Increased abdominal fat also raises your risk of cardiovascular diseases. This type of fat can lead to higher levels of inflammation, contributing to heart disease and stroke. Additionally, this fat can predispose you to metabolic syndrome, which includes high blood pressure, elevated blood sugar, and abnormal cholesterol levels. Metabolic syndrome also significantly increases your risk of heart disease, stroke, and diabetes.

Early intervention is pivotal in preventing these long-term health issues. By addressing metabolic changes as soon as they become apparent, you can take proactive steps to mitigate risks. Preventive measures include:

- Adopting a balanced diet rich in whole foods

- Engaging in regular physical activity

- Maintaining a healthy weight

These lifestyle adjustments can help regulate your metabolism and improve overall health. The benefits of early intervention extend beyond physical health. Taking control of your metabolism can also boost your confidence and emotional well-being, providing a sense of empowerment during a time of significant change.

Effective Diet Plans for Weight Management

You'll want to Incorporate nutrient-dense foods into your diet to maintain a healthy weight during menopause. Whole grains like quinoa and oats are excellent choices, as they are rich in fiber, which helps keep you full longer and provides essential vitamins and minerals. These grains can be a versatile addition to your meals, whether as a base for salads, a filling breakfast porridge, or a side dish. Lean proteins such as chicken, fish, and legumes are also vital; they support muscle maintenance and repair, which is essential, as muscle mass tends to decrease during menopause. Adding healthy fats from avocados, nuts, and olive oil can further enhance your diet. These fats help keep you satiated and support overall health by providing essential fatty acids and promoting heart health.

Mindful Eating

Portion control and mindful eating can significantly impact your weight-management efforts. Using smaller plates can help control portion sizes without leaving you feeling deprived. By visually filling a smaller plate, you can trick your brain into feeling satisfied with less food. Eating slowly and savoring each bite is another effective strategy—it allows your body time to signal fullness to your brain, reducing the likelihood of overeating. Pay close attention to your hunger and fullness cues. Before reaching for a snack or second helping, take a moment to assess whether you are truly hungry or just eating out of habit or boredom. Recognizing these cues can help you make more mindful eating choices and prevent unnecessary calorie intake.

Meal Planning

Meal planning and preparation can streamline your efforts to maintain a balanced diet. Creating a weekly meal plan ensures you have healthy meals and snacks readily available, reducing the temptation to reach for less nutritious options. Batch cooking and portioning meals for the week can save you time and effort, making it easier to stick to your dietary goals. Preparing healthy snack options, such as fresh fruits, vegetables, and nuts, can also support your weight management. These snacks provide essential nutrients and help curb hunger between meals, preventing overeating at main meals.

Several specific diet plans have been shown to support weight management during menopause. The Mediterranean diet, for example, emphasizes whole grains, lean proteins, healthy fats, and plenty of fruits and vegetables. This diet is rich in antioxidants and healthy fats, which can help reduce inflammation and support overall health. Another effective approach is a plant-based diet. By focusing on foods such as vegetables, fruits, legumes, nuts, and seeds, you can increase your fiber and essential nutrients intake while reducing the consumption of unhealthy fats and processed foods.

Intermittent Fasting

Intermittent fasting is another dietary approach that can impact metabolism and weight management. This method involves cycling between periods of eating and fasting. For women, intermittent fasting can work differently than for men due to hormonal fluctuations. Be sure to choose a fasting technique that aligns with your lifestyle and health needs. One popular method is the 16/8 technique, where you fast for 16 hours and eat during an 8-hour window. Another approach is the 5:2 technique, where you eat normally for 5 days and reduce calorie intake significantly on 2 non-consecutive days. Intermittent fasting can help regulate insulin levels, support weight loss, and improve metabolic health. However, always consider potential risks and medical conditions and consult a healthcare provider before starting any fasting regimen to ensure it's safe and appropriate for you.

Metabolic Confusion and Menopause

Metabolic confusion, also known as calorie shifting or calorie cycling, has gained attention as a potential strategy to support metabolism and manage weight during menopause.

What Is Metabolic Confusion?

Metabolic confusion is a dietary approach that involves alternating calorie intake between high- and low-calorie days. This pattern aims to "trick" the metabolism into staying more active rather than adapting to a consistent calorie deficit, which can lead to a slower metabolic rate over time. By preventing the body from getting used to one specific caloric intake, metabolic confusion can help women maintain a more efficient metabolic rate, which is particularly beneficial during menopause, when metabolism naturally slows down due to hormonal shifts.

The Science Behind Metabolic Confusion

During menopause, estrogen and progesterone levels decrease, which can cause a shift in body fat distribution and a reduction in lean muscle mass. These changes contribute to the slowdown in metabolism and often lead to weight gain, especially in the abdominal area. Metabolic confusion operates on the principle that changing calorie intake regularly keeps the body from entering a "starvation mode," where the metabolism adjusts downward to conserve energy.

Some studies suggest that metabolic confusion can improve metabolic flexibility—the body's ability to switch between burning carbohydrates and fats for energy—which can help with weight management and energy balance. This dietary approach contrasts with a traditional, consistent calorie-restricted diet, which can lead to plateaus when the metabolism slows to match the decreased intake.

How Metabolic Confusion Benefits Women in Menopause

- **Prevents metabolic slowdown:** One major challenge during menopause is slowing metabolism. By alternating between high- and low-calorie days, metabolic confusion can keep the metabolism more active, reducing the risk of the body adapting to a lower calorie intake.

- **Supports lean muscle mass:** Muscle mass naturally declines with age and menopause, and maintaining muscle is incredibly important for metabolic health. On higher-calorie days, women can focus on consuming more protein to support muscle repair and growth, helping to counter the muscle loss typically seen during menopause.

- **Reduces weight gain:** By keeping the body's metabolism more engaged, metabolic confusion can help women avoid the weight gain commonly associated with menopause, particularly the accumulation of visceral fat, which is linked to cardiovascular risk.

- **Promotes hormonal balance:** While it does not directly influence hormone levels, maintaining a healthy metabolism and weight can contribute to better hormonal balance. Reducing fat around the abdomen can improve insulin sensitivity and support overall hormonal health.

Implementing Metabolic Confusion During Menopause

You'll need to plan for alternating calorie intake when implementing metabolic confusion while ensuring nutritional needs are met, especially during menopause. Here are a few steps to follow:

1. **Calorie cycling:** Start by calculating your total daily energy expenditure (TDEE), which estimates how many calories your body needs daily. On high-calorie days, eat slightly above this number; on low-calorie days, reduce your intake by 15%–25%. For example, if your TDEE is 1,800 calories, a high-calorie day might be around 2,000–2,200 calories, and a low-calorie day around 1,300–1,500 calories.

2. **Protein focus:** On higher-calorie days, increase your intake of lean proteins such as chicken, fish, tofu, and legumes, which support muscle health and repair. Protein is particularly important during menopause to help offset the decline in muscle mass.

3. **Balance nutrients:** Ensure that both high- and low-calorie days include balanced meals with healthy fats, complex carbohydrates, and plenty of fiber. This will help stabilize blood sugar levels and support digestion, both of which are crucial during menopause.

4. **Exercise Integration:** To optimize the benefits of metabolic confusion, combine it with regular physical activity. Resistance training, in particular, helps to maintain muscle mass and further supports metabolic health. Aerobic activities like walking, cycling, and swimming can complement metabolic confusion by improving cardiovascular health.

Potential Downsides and Considerations

While metabolic confusion can be effective for some, it may not be suitable for everyone. Women who have a history of disordered eating or struggle with strict dietary regimens may find the constant calorie adjustments overwhelming. As with any diet, focusing on nutrient-dense foods and not just calorie counts is essential.

Some studies also suggest that individual metabolic responses vary widely, and while calorie cycling works for some, others may not experience significant differences compared to traditional calorie-restricted diets. Before starting any new dietary plan, consulting with a healthcare provider is recommended, especially during menopause, when specific nutritional needs may need to be addressed.

Metabolic confusion offers a flexible approach to managing weight and supporting metabolic health during menopause. By alternating calorie intake, women can avoid metabolic slowdown, support muscle retention, and reduce the risk of menopause-related weight gain. This approach, combined with a balanced diet and regular exercise, can be a valuable tool for women looking to maintain their health and vitality through menopause.

Exercise Routines for Menopausal Women

Exercise is a powerful tool for managing weight and overall health at any time, especially during menopause. Resistance training, in particular, offers numerous benefits. Building and maintaining muscle mass is essential, especially as muscle mass naturally declines with age. Resistance exercises such as weight lifting or using resistance bands help counteract this loss. As muscle mass increases, your metabolic rate also rises, allowing you to burn more calories even at rest. Additionally, resistance training effectively reduces body fat, helping to improve body composition and reduce the risk of obesity-related conditions. You can incorporate activities such as squats, lunges, and push-ups into your routine, providing a balanced approach to strength training.

Cardiovascular Exercises

Cardiovascular exercises are equally important for menopausal women. Activities like brisk walking, cycling, and swimming offer significant benefits for heart health and weight management. These exercises elevate your heart rate, improve cardiovascular fitness, and help you burn calories. Aim for at least 150 minutes of moderate-intensity exercise per week to reap the benefits, which can be broken down into manageable sessions, such as 30 minutes, 5 days a week. Cardiovascular exercises help maintain a healthy weight and reduce the risk of heart disease, which becomes more prevalent post-menopause. Engaging in activities you enjoy can make it easier to stick to a routine, whether you join a local cycling group or swimming club.

Flexibility and Balance

Flexibility and balance training play a vital role in overall fitness during menopause. Yoga is an excellent option for enhancing flexibility and reducing stress. The various poses and stretches improve joint mobility and muscle flexibility, while the deep-breathing techniques promote relaxation and mental clarity. Pilates, another effective form of exercise, focuses on core strength and balance. The controlled movements and exercises strengthen the abdominal muscles and improve posture. Simple balance exercises can also be beneficial, such as standing on one leg or using a balance board. These exercises help maintain stability and reduce the risk of falls, which is particularly important as bone density decreases.

Creating a sustainable and enjoyable exercise routine is key to long-term success. Finding activities you enjoy ensures that exercise becomes a regular and enjoyable part of your life. Whether it's dancing, hiking, or gardening, engaging in activities that are fun can make exercise feel less like a chore. Setting realistic and achievable goals is also important. Start with small, manageable targets and gradually increase the intensity and duration of your workouts. This approach helps you build confidence and ensures you are making steady progress. Simple activities can also add up over time. Consider taking the stairs instead of the elevator or walking during breaks.

Exercise Routine Checklist

- **Resistance training:** Include exercises such as weight lifting, resistance bands, squats, lunges, and push-ups.

- **Cardiovascular exercises:** Aim for moderate-intensity exercise such as brisk walking, cycling, or swimming.

- **Flexibility and balance training:** Practicing yoga, Pilates, and simple balance exercises like standing on one leg can improve flexibility and balance.

- **Sustainable routine:** Choose activities you enjoy, set realistic goals, and incorporate physical activity into your daily life.

Integrating these elements into your exercise routine allows you to effectively manage your weight and enhance your overall health during menopause. Consistency and enjoyment are beneficial to maintaining an active lifestyle that supports both physical and emotional well-being.

HIIT Workouts for Menopausal Women

High-intensity interval training (HIIT) has gained popularity as a highly effective workout for people of all ages, and it holds particular benefits for women going through menopause. As the body undergoes significant hormonal changes, including declines in estrogen and progesterone, many women experience weight gain, fatigue, loss of muscle mass, and a decrease in bone density. HIIT offers a time-efficient, adaptable, and effective way to combat these challenges and support overall health during menopause.

What Is HIIT?

HIIT involves short bursts of intense exercise followed by periods of rest or lower-intensity activity. These workouts typically last 20–30 minutes and can be adapted to various fitness levels. The intensity of the "work" phase is meant to challenge the cardiovascular system, boost metabolism, and burn calories efficiently. The rest periods allow recovery before diving into the next high-intensity interval.

The Science Behind HIIT and Menopause

Research suggests that HIIT workouts are particularly beneficial for menopausal women because of their impact on cardiovascular health, fat loss, muscle retention, and metabolic rate. Unlike traditional steady-state cardio, which can lead to a plateau in weight loss, HIIT continues to burn calories even after the workout ends due to the afterburn effect, also known as excess post-exercise oxygen consumption (EPOC).

Benefits of HIIT for Menopausal Women

- **Improves cardiovascular health:** The risk of heart disease increases during menopause due to a decrease in estrogen, which has a protective effect on the heart. HIIT has been shown to improve cardiovascular fitness by enhancing heart function and improving blood circulation. Studies suggest that HIIT may also reduce blood pressure and improve cholesterol levels, both of which are significant changes for menopausal women.

- **Increases fat loss and maintains lean muscle:** One major challenge of menopause is weight gain, particularly around the midsection. HIIT is highly effective at burning fat while preserving lean muscle mass, which is essential for keeping the metabolism active. Research shows HIIT workouts can help women lose more abdominal fat than moderate-intensity continuous training.

- **Boosts metabolism:** HIIT workouts stimulate both aerobic and anaerobic energy systems, leading to an increased metabolic rate that can last for hours after the workout is finished. This is particularly beneficial for menopausal women, as metabolism tends to slow down during this stage of life. A higher metabolic rate can help combat the weight gain often associated with menopause.

- **Supports bone health:** The decline in estrogen levels during menopause contributes to bone loss, putting women at greater risk for osteoporosis. HIIT, which includes weight-bearing exercises such as jumping, squatting, and lunging, helps to stimulate bone formation and maintain bone density. This can reduce the risk of fractures and support long-term skeletal health.

- **Enhances mood and reduces stress:** HIIT workouts trigger the release of endorphins, which are natural mood boosters. This is particularly important for menopausal women, who often experience mood swings, anxiety, and depression due to hormonal fluctuations. HIIT can also help reduce levels of the stress hormone cortisol, which is linked to fat storage, particularly around the abdomen.

HIIT Safety Considerations for Menopausal Women

While HIIT offers numerous benefits, it's important to approach it cautiously, particularly for women new to high-intensity workouts or with specific health concerns. Here are a few tips for safely incorporating HIIT into a fitness routine during menopause:

- **Start slow and progress gradually:** For those new to HIIT, you need to ease into the workouts. Begin with lower-intensity intervals and longer rest periods, gradually increasing the intensity and reducing the rest times as fitness improves.

- **Incorporate strength training:** Strength training is very beneficial for menopausal women, counteracting muscle loss and maintaining bone density. A well-rounded HIIT routine should include strength exercises such as bodyweight squats, lunges, push-ups, and resistance-based movements using weights or resistance bands.

- **Focus on recovery:** Recovery is just as important as the workout itself, especially for women going through menopause, who may be more prone to joint discomfort or injury. Ensure adequate rest between HIIT sessions and include active recovery activities like stretching, yoga, or walking on non-HIIT days.

- **Listen to your body:** Hormonal changes during menopause can cause fluctuations in energy levels, so it's important to listen to your body and adjust workouts accordingly. Some days, you might have the energy to push hard during HIIT, while other days might require moderation.

- **Consult a healthcare provider:** Before starting any new workout regimen, particularly one as intense as HIIT, you'll want to consult with a healthcare provider, especially if you have underlying health conditions like osteoporosis, heart disease, or joint issues.

Sample HIIT Workout for Menopausal Women

Here's a beginner-friendly HIIT workout designed for menopausal women that can be completed in about 20 minutes. Remember to warm up with light cardio and dynamic stretching before starting the workout.

Circuit

1. Jumping jacks: 30 seconds. (low-impact option: step jacks) Rest for 30 seconds.

2. Bodyweight squats: 30 seconds. Rest for 30 seconds.

3. Mountain climbers: 30 seconds. (low-impact option: slow climbers) Rest for 30 seconds.

4. Push-ups: 30 seconds. (can be done on knees or against a wall for modifications) Rest for 30 seconds.

5. High knees: 30 seconds. (low-impact option: march in place) Rest for 30 seconds.

Repeat circuit 3 times.

Cool Down

Stretch major muscle groups, holding each stretch for 20–30 seconds to promote flexibility and reduce muscle tension.

HIIT is an excellent workout option for menopausal women. It offers a range of health benefits, from improved cardiovascular fitness and fat loss to enhanced bone health and mood regulation. By incorporating HIIT into your fitness routines, you can address some of the key challenges of menopause, including weight gain, muscle loss, and reduced energy. With its time-efficient and adaptable structure, HIIT empowers women to stay active, healthy, and strong during this transitional phase of life.

GLP-1 Medications

Glucagon-like peptide-1 (GLP-1) is a significant hormone in regulating appetite and blood sugar levels. It is naturally produced in the gut and released in response to food intake. GLP-1 helps slow down gastric emptying, promotes the feeling of fullness, and enhances insulin secretion while inhibiting glucagon release. These actions collectively help control blood sugar levels and reduce appetite, making GLP-1 a valuable target for weight-management medications, especially for women experiencing menopause-related weight gain.

GLP-1 medications, such as semaglutide, are designed to mimic the effects of the natural hormone. They work by binding to GLP-1 receptors in the brain and gut, promoting a sense of satiety and reducing hunger. This helps you eat less and feel satisfied with smaller portions, leading to weight loss. Additionally, GLP-1 medications improve insulin sensitivity and help lower blood sugar levels, which is particularly beneficial if you're dealing with insulin resistance, a common issue during menopause. These medications can be a powerful tool in managing weight, especially when combined with a balanced diet and regular exercise.

GLP-1 Benefits and Risks

However, like any medication, GLP-1 treatments come with their risks and benefits. The benefits are clear: significant weight loss, improved blood sugar control, and reduced appetite. Many women find that these medications help them regain control over their eating habits and achieve a healthier weight. The positive effects on blood sugar levels also mean a reduced risk of developing type 2 diabetes, which is a significant concern during menopause. However, you need to be aware of the potential side effects. Common side effects include nausea, vomiting, and diarrhea, particularly when first starting the medication. These symptoms often subside as your body adjusts. There are also more serious risks, such as pancreatitis and gallbladder disease, although these are less common. Understanding these risks can help you make an informed decision about whether GLP-1 medications are right for you.

You cannot start GLP-1 medications before discussing it with your doctor—they can help determine whether this treatment is suitable for your specific situation, considering your medical history, current health status, and any other medications you might be taking. They can also monitor your progress and manage any side effects that may arise. Open communication with your doctor ensures that you receive personalized advice and a treatment plan tailored to your needs. It's also an opportunity to discuss your concerns and explore alternative options if GLP-1 medications are not the best fit for you.

Before starting any new medication, you need to have a comprehensive understanding of how it works and what to expect. Your doctor can explain the mechanism of GLP-1 medications in detail, helping you understand how they will interact with your body. They can also provide guidance on the proper dosage and administration, ensuring that you start on the right foot. Monitoring your progress is equally important. Regular follow-ups with your healthcare provider allow for adjustments to your treatment plan as needed and ensure that you achieve the best possible outcomes while minimizing potential risks.

Incorporating GLP-1 medications into your weight-management strategy can be a game-changer. These medications offer a science-backed approach to appetite suppression and weight loss, addressing some of the unique challenges faced during menopause. By working closely with your healthcare provider, you can better understand the complexities of this treatment and find a solution that supports your overall health and well-being. Understanding the potential risks and benefits and having a clear plan for monitoring and adjustment can make all the difference in your weight-management journey.

Monitoring and Maintaining a Healthy Weight

Tracking your progress is necessary for effective weight management, especially during menopause. Keeping a food and exercise journal can provide valuable insights into your habits and patterns. By writing down what you eat and how much you exercise, you can identify areas for improvement and celebrate your successes, a practice that lets you see the direct correlation between your efforts and results. Numerous apps and tools are available to help you monitor your calorie intake and physical activity. These apps can simplify the process, offering features like barcode scanning for food items and syncing with fitness trackers. Regularly measuring your weight and body composition can also keep you on track. While the scale provides a quick snapshot, body composition measurements, such as body fat percentage, offer you a more comprehensive view of your progress.

Setting realistic goals is another key component of successful weight management. Focusing on gradual weight loss, such as 1–2 pounds per week, is both achievable and sustainable. Rapid weight loss can often lead to yo-yo dieting and is generally not healthy. Start by setting short-term goals, like losing 5 pounds or increasing your daily steps by 1,000. These smaller milestones can provide immediate gratification and keep you motivated. Setting long-term goals, such as reaching a specific weight or maintaining a new lifestyle, offers a broader vision to work toward. Celebrating small milestones is essential. When you reach these goals, treat yourself to a new book, a spa day, or a fun outing with friends. Positive reinforcement makes the journey enjoyable and keeps you motivated.

Professional guidance can provide the expertise and support you need to navigate weight management successfully. Consulting a registered dietitian or nutritionist can offer personalized dietary advice that addresses your needs and preferences. These professionals can help you create a balanced meal plan that aligns with your weight loss goals. Working with a personal trainer can further enhance your efforts. Trainers can design exercise routines that suit your fitness level and help you progress safely and effectively. Seeking medical advice for underlying health issues affecting weight is also important. Conditions such as thyroid disorders or insulin resistance can hinder weight loss. A healthcare provider can diagnose and treat these issues, ensuring that your efforts are not in vain.

Staying Motivated

Maintaining motivation is often one of the biggest challenges in weight management. Finding a workout buddy or a support group can provide the accountability and encouragement you need to stay on track. Sharing your journey with others can make the process more enjoyable and less isolating. Keeping a positive mindset and focusing on overall health, not just weight, can also sustain your motivation. Remember that weight is just one aspect of health. Improved energy levels, better sleep, and enhanced mood are equally important progress indicators. You need to be flexible with your goals and adjust plans as needed. Life is unpredictable, and setbacks are normal. The key is to adapt and keep moving forward rather than give up entirely.

By tracking your progress, setting realistic goals, seeking professional guidance, and maintaining motivation, you can effectively manage your weight during menopause. These strategies provide a comprehensive approach to weight management, ensuring that you stay on track and achieve your goals.

This chapter has explored various strategies for managing weight and metabolism during menopause. From understanding metabolic changes to creating effective diet plans and exercise routines, these tools can help you confidently navigate this phase. In the next chapter, we will explore hormone replacement therapy in detail, examining its role in alleviating menopausal symptoms through the replenishment of diminishing hormone levels.

Chapter 6:

Hormone Replacement

Therapy (HRT)

Imagine sitting in your living room, flipping through old photo albums. Each picture brings back memories of feeling more like yourself—energetic, confident, and comfortable in your skin. Now, menopause has brought a slew of symptoms that seem to have hijacked your life. You've heard about Hormone replacement therapy (HRT) but aren't sure if it's right for you. This chapter aims to demystify HRT, providing the information you'll need to make an informed decision.

Introduction to HRT

Hormone replacement therapy, commonly known as HRT, is a treatment designed to relieve menopausal symptoms by replenishing the hormones your body no longer produces in sufficient quantities. The primary hormones involved in HRT are estrogen and progesterone. During your reproductive years, these hormones work harmoniously to regulate your menstrual cycle, maintain bone density, and support various bodily functions. As menopause approaches, the levels of these hormones decline. Symptoms like hot flashes, night sweats, mood swings, and vaginal dryness become prevalent. The primary purpose of HRT is to restore hormonal balance, thereby alleviating these symptoms and improving your quality of life.

Determining who might benefit from HRT involves considering various factors. Women who experience severe menopausal symptoms that significantly impact their daily lives are prime candidates. Hot flashes, night sweats, and sleep disturbances can be debilitating, affecting your ability to function at work and enjoy social activities. HRT can provide much-needed relief, allowing you to reclaim your life. Additionally, women who are at high risk for osteoporosis can also benefit from HRT. Estrogen plays a significant role in maintaining bone density, and its decline can lead to weakened bones and an increased risk of fractures. HRT can help mitigate this risk by preserving bone strength.

However, not everyone is a suitable candidate for HRT. Women with a history of breast cancer, blood clots, or certain cardiovascular conditions should approach HRT with caution. Discussing your medical history and current health status with your healthcare provider is important to determine whether HRT is right for you. The decision to start HRT should be based on a careful evaluation of the benefits and risks tailored to your specific needs and circumstances.

Reflection Section: Is HRT Right for You?

Reflect on the following questions to help determine whether HRT might be a suitable option for you:

- How severe are your menopausal symptoms, and how do they affect your daily life?

- Do you have a history of osteoporosis or other conditions that might benefit from HRT?

- What are your personal and family medical histories— in particular, breast cancer and cardiovascular diseases?

- What are your preferences regarding the form of HRT (oral, transdermal, topical, or vaginal)?

- Have you discussed HRT's potential benefits and risks with your healthcare provider?

By carefully considering these questions and consulting with your healthcare provider, you can make an informed decision about whether HRT is the right choice for managing your menopausal symptoms.

Bioidentical Hormones: Myths and Facts

Bioidentical hormones have become a popular topic among women seeking relief from menopausal symptoms. But what exactly are they? Bioidentical hormones are chemically identical to the hormones produced by your body and are often derived from plant sources like soy and yams. This contrasts with synthetic hormones, which may have similar effects but different chemical structures. The term "bioidentical" means that these hormones match what your body naturally produces, which is why many believe they are more effective and safer than synthetic options.

However, several myths surround bioidentical hormones. One common misconception is that because they are "natural," they are entirely risk-free. This is not true. While bioidentical hormones are derived from natural sources, they still require processing and compounding, which can introduce risks. Another myth is that bioidentical hormones are inherently more effective than synthetic hormones. Scientific studies have shown that both types can be equally effective in managing menopausal symptoms. The idea that bioidentical hormones do not require medical supervision is also false. Like any hormone therapy, bioidentical hormones need careful monitoring to avoid potential side effects and ensure optimal benefits.

Scientific evidence supports the use of bioidentical hormones, but it's essential to understand the nuances. Studies comparing bioidentical and synthetic hormones have found both to be effective in relieving menopausal symptoms like hot flashes, night sweats, and mood swings. However, some research indicates that bioidentical hormones might have a better safety profile, particularly regarding breast cancer risk. For instance, a study published in JAMA found that modern hormone therapies, including bioidentical hormones, are safer than older formulations. The Women's Health Initiative, a landmark study, previously linked hormone therapy with increased risks of breast cancer and stroke. However, newer studies show that using bioidentical hormones and lower doses of estrogen and progesterone can mitigate these risks.

Choosing bioidentical hormones involves careful consideration and consultation with a healthcare provider. Your doctor can help you understand whether bioidentical hormones are suitable based on your medical history and current symptoms. Compounded bioidentical hormones are not FDA-approved, meaning their quality can vary. Therefore, you need to choose a reputable pharmacy that follows strict guidelines and uses high-quality ingredients.

Monitoring and adjusting the dosage is another critical aspect of using bioidentical hormones. Regular follow-ups with your healthcare provider are essential to track your symptoms and hormone levels. Checkups allow for timely adjustments to your treatment plan, ensuring you receive the optimal dosage for your needs. Bioidentical hormones can offer significant relief from menopausal symptoms, but they are not a one-size-fits-all solution. Personalized care and vigilant monitoring are key to achieving the best outcomes.

Checklist: What to Ask Your Healthcare Provider

Before starting bioidentical hormone therapy, consider asking your healthcare provider the following questions:

- What are bioidentical hormones' potential benefits and risks for my specific symptoms?

- How often will I need to have my hormone levels checked?

- Can you recommend a reputable compounding pharmacy?

- What are the signs that my dosage might need adjusting?

- Are there any lifestyle changes I should make to complement my hormone therapy?

By understanding the complexities of bioidentical hormones, you can make informed decisions about your treatment options. This knowledge empowers you to take control of your health and well-being during menopause.

Benefits and Risks of HRT

HRT can significantly alleviate the symptoms of menopause, making day-to-day life more manageable. One of the most immediate benefits is the reduction in hot flashes and night sweats. These sudden waves of heat and perspiration can disrupt your daily activities as well as your sleep. HRT helps stabilize your body's temperature regulation, making these episodes less frequent and less severe. Improved sleep quality is another fundamental benefit. You can achieve deeper, more restful sleep with fewer night sweats and a more balanced hormonal environment. Improvement in sleep can lead to better overall health, increasing your energy levels and mood. Vaginal dryness and discomfort, common symptoms of menopause, are also alleviated with HRT. Estrogen therapy helps maintain the thickness and elasticity of vaginal tissues, reducing dryness and making sexual activity more comfortable.

Beyond symptom relief, HRT offers several long-term health benefits that can enhance your quality of life. One of the most significant advantages is the prevention of osteoporosis and bone fractures. Estrogen plays a major role in maintaining bone density; its decline during menopause can lead to weakened bones. HRT helps preserve bone strength, reducing the risk of fractures. Studies have also shown that HRT can potentially reduce the risk of colorectal cancer. The mechanisms are not fully understood, but it is believed that estrogen helps protect against the development of cancerous cells in the colon and rectum. Additionally, HRT can improve cardiovascular health for certain individuals. Estrogen has a protective effect on the heart, helping to maintain healthy blood vessels and reduce the risk of heart disease. However, this benefit is more pronounced in younger postmenopausal women and those who start HRT soon after menopause.

Despite these benefits, HRT is not without risks and side effects. One of the most concerning risks is the increased likelihood of breast cancer. This risk varies depending on the type and duration of HRT. For instance, combined estrogen-progesterone therapy has been associated with a higher risk than estrogen-only therapy. Another significant risk is the potential for blood clots and stroke. Estrogen can increase the tendency for blood to clot, leading to conditions such as deep vein thrombosis (DVT) and pulmonary embolism. This risk is particularly relevant for women who smoke or have a history of blood clots. Common side effects of HRT include bloating, nausea, and headaches. These symptoms often subside as your body adjusts to the therapy, but they can be bothersome initially. It's important to discuss any side effects with your healthcare provider to determine whether adjustments to your treatment plan are needed.

Weighing the benefits and risks of HRT is an important step in deciding whether this therapy is right for you. You need to carefully consider individual risk factors, such as a family history of cancer or personal health history. For example, if you have a family history of breast cancer, you may need to approach HRT with caution. Regular health checkups and monitoring are essential while on HRT. These appointments allow your healthcare provider to track your progress, monitor for any adverse effects, and make necessary adjustments to your treatment plan. Personalization of HRT is key to minimizing risks. Starting with the lowest effective dose and gradually adjusting as needed can help you achieve the desired benefits while reducing potential side effects. Your healthcare provider will work closely with you to customize your HRT regimen, ensuring it meets your specific needs and health profile.

Customizing HRT

Every woman experiences menopause differently, and the same applies to HRT. Personalized treatment plans are a must for effectively managing your symptoms. Several factors influence the choice of HRT, including your age, the severity of your symptoms, and your health history. Younger women who enter menopause prematurely might require different dosages and types of hormones compared with those who reach menopause at the average age. The severity of symptoms, such as hot flashes and night sweats, also plays a significant role. Women with milder symptoms might benefit from lower doses, while those with more severe symptoms might need higher doses. Starting with the lowest effective dose is always recommended; this minimizes potential side effects while still providing relief. As your body adjusts, your healthcare provider can make necessary adjustments to optimize your treatment.

The types of hormones and combinations used in HRT are designed to meet specific needs. Estrogen-only therapy is often prescribed for women who have had a hysterectomy, as they do not need progesterone to protect the uterine lining. For those who still have their uterus, combined estrogen-progesterone therapy is usually recommended to reduce the risk of endometrial cancer. As previously discussed, bioidentical hormones, which are chemically identical to those produced by your body, offer another option. These hormones are often perceived to be more natural and better tolerated, although they require careful monitoring and precise dosing.

Administration Methods

Administration methods for HRT vary, and each has its advantages and disadvantages.

- Oral tablets are convenient and easy to take but pass through the digestive system, affecting their absorption and increasing the risk of blood clots.

- Transdermal patches deliver hormones directly into the bloodstream through the skin, offering a steady release and reducing the risk of clotting.

- Topical gels and creams are applied to the skin and absorbed into the bloodstream, providing flexibility in dosing.

- Vaginal rings and suppositories are specifically designed to address vaginal symptoms, delivering hormones directly to the affected area.

Matching the administration method to your preferences and lifestyle is crucial for adherence and effectiveness. For example, a patch or ring might be more suitable if you prefer not to take daily medication. Your healthcare provider can help you determine the best method based on your needs.

Adjusting and monitoring your HRT is an ongoing process. Regular follow-ups with your healthcare provider are essential to track your symptoms and ensure the treatment works effectively. Monitoring symptoms and side effects allows for timely adjustments to your dosage or administration method. For instance, if you experience side effects like bloating or headaches, your provider might lower your dose or switch you to a different form of HRT. Routine health checkups, including blood tests and bone density scans, are important for monitoring your overall health while on HRT. These tests can detect any potential issues early, allowing for prompt intervention.

Regular communication with your healthcare provider ensures that your treatment remains effective and safe. This collaboration allows personalized adjustments catering to your unique needs and circumstances. By staying proactive and engaged in your treatment plan, you can achieve better symptom management and improve your quality of life. The goal is to find a balance that alleviates your symptoms while minimizing risks, allowing you to navigate menopause with confidence and ease.

Discussing HRT With Your Healthcare Provider

Preparing for your appointment to discuss HRT can significantly affect the outcome. Start by making a comprehensive list of your symptoms and concerns. Note when they started, their frequency, and how they impact your daily life. Having a detailed account will give your healthcare provider a clear picture of your situation. Gather your personal and family medical history, focusing on conditions like breast cancer, heart disease, and osteoporosis. You'll need this information to assess the risks and benefits of HRT for you. Preparing questions in advance can also help you make the most of your appointment. Think about what you want to know and what concerns you have regarding HRT.

Be sure to ask the right questions when you meet with your healthcare provider. Start by inquiring about the benefits and risks of HRT for your specific situation. Each woman's experience with menopause is unique, and understanding how HRT can help you is essential. Ask about the different types of HRT available and which one best suits you. Understanding your options, whether it's oral tablets, patches, or creams, can help you make an informed decision. Another question is how the effectiveness and side effects of the treatment will be monitored. Regular checkups and adjustments are often necessary, and knowing what to expect can help you stay on track.

Discussing alternatives to HRT is also important. While HRT can be highly effective, it's not the only option for managing menopausal symptoms. Nonhormonal treatments, such as antidepressants for mood swings or medications for hot flashes, could be suitable alternatives. Lifestyle changes, such as improving your diet, increasing physical activity, and practicing stress-reduction techniques, can also significantly impact your symptoms. Natural remedies, such as herbal supplements, can offer relief for some women. Integrative approaches that combine conventional and alternative treatments can provide a comprehensive strategy for managing menopause. Being open to discussing these alternatives with your healthcare provider can help you find the best approach for your needs.

Building a collaborative relationship with your healthcare provider is important for successfully managing menopausal symptoms. Be open about your preferences and concerns. If you have reservations about HRT or prefer natural remedies, communicate this to your provider. Regularly update them on any changes in your symptoms or side effects. Keeping an open line of communication ensures that your treatment plan can be adjusted as needed. Working together with your healthcare provider allows you to find treatment that meets your unique needs. This partnership can make a significant difference in your menopause experience, helping you through this phase of life with greater ease and confidence.

Checklist: Preparing for Your Appointment

1. **List of symptoms:** Note when symptoms started, their frequency, and their impact on daily life.

2. **Medical history:** Gather personal and family medical history, focusing on conditions like breast cancer and osteoporosis.

3. **Questions to ask:**

    o   What are the benefits and risks of HRT for my specific situation?

o What types of HRT are available, and which one is best for me?

o How will we monitor the effectiveness and side effects of the treatment?

4. **Discussing alternatives:** Be open to nonhormonal treatments, lifestyle changes, natural remedies, and integrative approaches.

5. **Building a relationship:** Be honest about preferences and concerns, update on changes, and work together to adjust treatment plans.

By preparing for your appointment, asking the right questions, discussing all available options, and building a collaborative relationship with your healthcare provider, you can make informed decisions about your menopausal treatment. This proactive approach empowers you to take control of your health and well-being.

In the next chapter, we will explore the digestive system and how menopause affects it, providing strategies and solutions to manage symptoms and maintain overall digestive health.

Chapter 7:

Digestive Health

For many women over 50, digestive issues can become all too common during menopause. Have you ever sat down to enjoy a meal with friends, only to be interrupted by a sudden bout of very uncomfortable acid reflux? Then you know. The hormonal shifts that occur during this time significantly impact your digestive system, often leading to discomfort and disrupting your daily life. Understanding these changes and how to manage them is essential for maintaining your overall health and well-being.

Digestive Changes During Menopause

As you go through menopause, you'll find that hormonal fluctuations play a significant role in how your body processes food. Decreased estrogen levels slow your digestive transit time, making it harder for your body to move food through the gastrointestinal tract efficiently. This slowdown can lead to constipation, as waste materials linger longer in the colon, absorbing more water and becoming harder to pass. Estrogen also affects the production of bile, which helps digest fats. With lower estrogen levels, bile can become more concentrated, increasing the risk of gallbladder issues such as gallstones. Hormonal changes during menopause also increase the risk of gastrointestinal problems like irritable bowel syndrome (IBS). Women who already suffer from IBS may find that their symptoms worsen during menopause. The impact on gut motility and bowel regularity can lead to a range of uncomfortable symptoms, from bloating and gas to constipation and diarrhea.

Common digestive symptoms during menopause include bloating and gas, making you uncomfortable and self-conscious. This bloating often occurs because the slowing of digestive transit allows for more gas to build up in the intestines. Constipation is another frequent complaint resulting from hormonal changes and decreased physical activity that often accompanies aging. Acid reflux and heartburn can also become more prevalent. As estrogen levels drop, the lower esophageal sphincter, which normally prevents stomach acid from rising into the esophagus, may weaken, resulting in that familiar burning sensation. You might also notice changes in your appetite and food sensitivities. Foods you once enjoyed without issue might now cause you discomfort or indigestion. These changes can be frustrating and confusing, but understanding their root causes can help you manage them more effectively.

The Impact of Stress on Digestion

Stress is another significant factor that can exacerbate digestive issues during menopause. The hormonal fluctuations you experience can trigger stress, which, in turn, affects your gut function. Stress can alter the gut-brain axis, a complex communication network between your brain and digestive system. When stressed, your body releases hormones such as cortisol, which can slow down digestion and increase the likelihood of constipation and bloating. Anxiety can also lead to digestive discomfort, as it often causes you to eat quickly or choose less healthy foods, both of which can upset your stomach. Managing stress is necessary for maintaining digestive health during menopause. Techniques such as mindfulness meditation, deep-breathing exercises, and yoga can help calm your mind and improve gut function. Regular physical activity, even something as simple as a daily walk, can also help reduce stress and improve digestion.

Not managing these digestive issues can lead to long-term health risks. Chronic constipation can cause hemorrhoids, anal fissures, and even fecal impaction, a severe condition in which hard stool gets stuck in the intestines. Persistent acid reflux can lead to gastroesophageal reflux disease (GERD), which can cause inflammation and damage to the esophagus. Unmanaged digestive issues can also affect your overall health and quality of life. When you're constantly dealing with discomfort, enjoying social activities, maintaining a healthy diet, and getting enough physical exercise can be challenging. Early intervention and regular monitoring are needed to prevent these complications. Consulting a gastrointestinal specialist can help you develop a personalized plan to manage your symptoms and maintain your digestive health.

Reflection Section: Digestive Health Journal

Keeping a digestive health journal can help you identify patterns and triggers for your symptoms. Every day, write what you eat, any digestive symptoms you experience, and any stressors or activities that might have influenced your digestion. Over time, this journal can provide valuable insights into how your diet, lifestyle, and stress levels impact your digestive health. A journal can also be a helpful tool when discussing your symptoms with a healthcare provider.

Understanding the digestive changes during menopause and taking proactive steps to manage them can significantly improve your quality of life. Addressing these issues head-on, you can maintain a healthy digestive system and enjoy your meals without discomfort.

Diet and Digestive Health: Foods to Include

Fiber-Rich Foods

Incorporating fiber-rich foods into your diet is one of the most effective ways to support digestive health during menopause. Fiber is vital in maintaining bowel regularity and preventing constipation, a common issue as your digestive transit time slows down. Whole grains like oats and quinoa are excellent sources of fiber and will help keep you regular and provide essential nutrients such as vitamins and minerals. Including fruits such as apples and berries in your diet can further boost your fiber intake. Apples contain soluble fiber, which helps soften stool and ease its passage through the intestines. Berries, rich in antioxidants, support overall gut health by reducing inflammation and promoting a healthy gut microbiome. Vegetables like broccoli and leafy greens offer a double benefit: They are high in fiber and packed with vitamins that support your digestive system. Legumes, including beans and lentils, are another fantastic source of fiber; they also provide protein and essential nutrients, making them a versatile addition to your meals.

Anti-Inflammatory Foods

Anti-inflammatory foods support digestive health, particularly during menopause, when inflammation can exacerbate symptoms. Turmeric, known for its active compound curcumin, has powerful anti-inflammatory properties. Adding turmeric to your recipes is an easy way to reduce inflammation in the digestive tract and improve overall gut health. Ginger is another anti-inflammatory food that offers digestive benefits. It can help alleviate nausea, reduce bloating, and improve digestion. You can incorporate ginger into your diet by adding fresh ginger to smoothies, teas, or stir-fries. Omega-3 fatty acids in fatty fish like salmon are also beneficial. These healthy fats help reduce inflammation and support the lining of the digestive tract. Including berries in your diet provides antioxidants that help combat oxidative stress, which can negatively impact your digestive health. The combination of fiber and antioxidants in berries makes them a powerful ally in helping you maintain a healthy gut.

Hydration

Staying hydrated is fundamental for maintaining digestive health. Drinking plenty of water throughout the day helps keep your digestive system running smoothly. Water aids in breaking down food and absorbing nutrients, and it also helps soften stool, making it easier to pass. Try to drink at least eight glasses of water a day. Herbal teas, such as peppermint and chamomile, can also support digestion. Peppermint tea helps relax the gastrointestinal tract muscles, reducing symptoms like bloating and gas. Chamomile tea has calming properties that help soothe digestive systems and reduce inflammation. Both options are caffeine-free, making them excellent choices for hydration without the risk of triggering digestive discomfort.

Planning meals that support digestive health involves creating balanced meals with fiber, protein, and healthy fats. Start your day with a breakfast with whole grains and fruits, such as oatmeal topped with berries and a sprinkle of flaxseeds. Consider a salad with leafy greens, beans, and a light vinaigrette for lunch. Including a source of lean protein, such as grilled chicken or tofu, can make the meal more satisfying. Dinner can feature a variety of vegetables, a serving of fatty fish like salmon, and a side of quinoa. Avoiding large, heavy meals can help you prevent digestive discomfort. Opt for smaller, frequent meals throughout the day to avoid overloading your digestive system. This approach also helps maintain stable blood sugar levels and provides you with a steady energy supply.

Probiotic-Rich Foods

Incorporating probiotic-rich foods, such as yogurt and kefir, can further enhance your digestive health. Probiotics are beneficial bacteria that support a healthy gut microbiome. Yogurt contains live cultures that help balance the bacteria in your gut, improving digestion and boosting your immune system. Kefir, a fermented milk drink, is another excellent source of probiotics. Including these foods in your diet can help you maintain a healthy balance of gut bacteria, reducing the risk of digestive issues like bloating, gas, and constipation. Fermented foods such as sauerkraut and kimchi also offer probiotic benefits and can be a flavorful addition to your meals.

Focusing on fiber-rich foods, anti-inflammatory ingredients, proper hydration, and balanced meals can support digestive health during menopause. These dietary changes can help alleviate symptoms and improve overall well-being, allowing you to enjoy your meals without discomfort.

Managing Bloating and Digestive Discomfort

You might find yourself frequently dealing with bloating and digestive discomfort during menopause. Identifying foods that trigger these symptoms is often the first step in managing them effectively. Keeping a food diary can help you spot patterns and pinpoint specific culprits. Every time you eat, jot down what you consumed and note any symptoms that follow. Good recordkeeping can reveal common triggers such as dairy, gluten, and high-fat foods. For instance, you might notice that a bowl of ice cream leads to bloating or that bread causes stomach cramps. An elimination diet can further refine your understanding. You can observe how your body reacts by removing suspected foods from your diet for a period and then reintroducing them one at a time. This process helps identify specific foods contributing to your discomfort, allowing you to make informed dietary choices.

Making lifestyle changes can also significantly reduce bloating and digestive discomfort. Eating slowly and chewing your food thoroughly can make a big difference. When you eat quickly, you tend to swallow air along with your food, which often leads to gas and bloating. Taking the time to chew properly aids in digestion and allows your stomach to signal fullness, helping you avoid overeating. Another simple yet effective change is to avoid carbonated beverages. These drinks introduce gas into your digestive system, which can exacerbate bloating. Opt for still water or herbal teas instead. Regular physical activity is another powerful tool. Exercise promotes gut motility, helping food move through your digestive tract more efficiently. Even a short daily walk can stimulate your intestines and reduce the likelihood of constipation and bloating.

Natural Remedies for Digestion

Natural remedies can offer relief from bloating and digestive discomfort. Peppermint oil capsules are known for their ability to relax the gastrointestinal tract muscles, reducing symptoms like bloating and gas. Taking these capsules before meals can help prevent discomfort. Ginger, whether in tea form or as a supplement, can also be beneficial. It has anti-inflammatory properties and aids digestion, making it a helpful remedy for nausea and bloating. Fennel seeds are another natural option. They have carminative properties, meaning they help expel gas from the digestive tract. Chewing a few fennel seeds after a meal can help reduce bloating. Digestive enzyme supplements can also be helpful. These supplements aid in breaking down food, making it easier for your body to absorb nutrients and reducing the risk of digestive discomfort. They can be particularly useful if you have trouble digesting certain foods, like dairy or high-fiber vegetables.

Sometimes, despite your best efforts, you might need to do more than make lifestyle changes and take natural remedies. In such cases, you should seek medical intervention. Consulting a gastroenterologist can provide you with a better understanding of your digestive issues. A specialist can perform tests to rule out more serious conditions and offer targeted treatments. Medications like antispasmodics can help reduce intestinal cramps and discomfort, while proton pump inhibitors can manage acid reflux and heartburn by reducing stomach acid production. You should get regular medical checkups to monitor your digestive health, especially if you experience severe or persistent symptoms. Early intervention can prevent minor issues from becoming more serious, ensuring you maintain a good quality of life.

Managing bloating and digestive discomfort involves a multifaceted approach. You can take control of your digestive health by identifying trigger foods, making lifestyle changes, using natural remedies, and seeking medical intervention when necessary. Each step brings you closer to a more comfortable and enjoyable daily life.

Probiotics and Gut Health

Probiotics are live micro-organisms that offer numerous health benefits, particularly for your digestive system. These beneficial bacteria are pivotal in maintaining a balanced gut microbiome for proper digestion and overall health. The gut microbiome is a complex community of bacteria, fungi, and other microbes that live in your digestive tract. When in balance, these micro-organisms help break down food, absorb nutrients, and protect against harmful pathogens. Common strains of probiotics include *Lactobacillus* and *Bifidobacterium*, each offering specific benefits. Lactobacillus strains are known for breaking down lactose, the sugar found in dairy, and producing lactic acid, which helps prevent harmful bacteria from colonizing the gut. Bifidobacterium strains effectively alleviate digestive issues like IBS and promote a healthy immune response.

Natural sources of probiotics are readily available in many fermented foods. Yogurt is the most well-known probiotic-rich food. It contains live cultures that help replenish the beneficial bacteria in your gut, improving digestion and boosting your immune system. Kefir, a fermented milk drink, is another excellent source of probiotics. It has a tangy taste and a higher probiotic content than yogurt. Including these foods in your diet can help you maintain a healthy balance of gut bacteria. Sauerkraut and kimchi, both fermented vegetables, are rich in probiotics and can add a flavorful twist to your meals. Miso and tempeh, fermented soybean products, offer plant-based sources of probiotics. These foods support gut health and provide essential nutrients like protein and vitamins. If you find it challenging to get enough probiotics from food alone, probiotic supplements are a convenient option. These supplements come in various forms, including capsules, tablets, and powders, making incorporating them into your daily routine effortless.

Prebiotics are equally important; they are nondigestible fibers that feed the beneficial bacteria in your gut. Think of prebiotics as the fertilizer for your gut's garden, helping probiotics thrive. Foods rich in prebiotics include garlic, onions, bananas, and asparagus. Garlic and onions are versatile ingredients that you can add to various dishes, providing flavor and prebiotic benefits. Bananas are convenient snacks that can be easily incorporated into smoothies or cereals. Asparagus, often enjoyed as a side dish, is another excellent source of prebiotics. Combining prebiotics with probiotics, often called synbiotics, can optimize gut health. This combination ensures that the beneficial bacteria have the nutrients they need to grow and flourish, enhancing their positive effects on your digestive system.

You'll want to consider several factors when choosing a probiotic supplement to ensure you get the most benefit. Strain specificity is crucial, as different strains offer different health benefits. For example, Lactobacillus rhamnosus GG is known for its ability to reduce the duration of diarrhea, while Bifidobacterium longum helps alleviate symptoms of IBS. The colony-forming unit (CFU) count indicates the number of live micro-organisms in each dose. A higher CFU count is generally more effective, but finding a balance that suits your needs is essential. The delivery method is another important factor. Some supplements are designed to survive stomach acid and reach the intestines, where they are most effective. Consulting with a healthcare provider can help you choose the right supplement for your specific needs. They can provide guidance on the appropriate strains and dosages based on your digestive health issues. Reading labels carefully and understanding product claims can also help you make an informed choice.

Incorporating probiotics and prebiotics into your diet can significantly improve your digestive health, particularly during menopause. These beneficial bacteria help balance your gut microbiome, reduce digestive discomfort, and support overall well-being. By choosing the right foods and supplements, you can take proactive steps to maintain a healthy digestive system and enjoy a better quality of life.

The next chapter will explore cardiovascular health, discussing how to maintain a healthy heart during and after menopause.

Chapter 8:

Cardiovascular Health

It's a lovely afternoon, and you're enjoying a moment of solitude, sipping tea and reading a book, when a sudden tightness grips your chest. You pause, trying to catch your breath, and a wave of dizziness washes over you. These moments can be frightening and are all too familiar for many women experiencing menopause. The hormonal changes during this phase significantly impact cardiovascular health, making understanding and addressing these risks essential.

Understanding Cardiovascular Risks in Menopause

Hormonal changes during menopause have a tremendous impact on your cardiovascular system. Estrogen declines during menopause and is vital in protecting your heart and blood vessels. Before menopause, estrogen helps maintain the flexibility and health of your blood vessels, promoting good circulation and preventing plaque buildup. This hormone also keeps your cholesterol levels in check by increasing high-density lipoprotein (HDL) cholesterol, which is often referred to as "healthy" cholesterol, and reducing low-density lipoprotein (LDL) cholesterol, known as "bad" cholesterol. As estrogen levels decline, these protective effects wane, leading to an increased risk of cardiovascular diseases.

The decline in estrogen during menopause affects your blood vessels and arterial health. Estrogen helps maintain the elasticity of your arteries, allowing them to expand and contract effortlessly with each heartbeat. Without sufficient estrogen, your arteries can become less flexible, increasing your blood pressure and elevating your risk of developing atherosclerosis, a hardening and narrowing of the arteries due to plaque buildup. These changes can significantly impact your cardiovascular health, making it more challenging for your heart to pump blood effectively throughout your body. Additionally, the drop in estrogen levels can lead to unfavorable changes in your cholesterol levels, increasing the risk of heart disease and stroke.

Hypertension, or high blood pressure, forces your heart to work harder to pump blood, increasing the risk of heart attacks and strokes. Atherosclerosis is another significant risk, characterized by the buildup of fatty deposits in your arteries, which restricts blood flow and may lead to serious cardiovascular events. The reduction in estrogen also contributes to dyslipidemia, a condition marked by abnormal cholesterol levels, further elevating the risk of heart disease. These combined factors make cardiovascular health a critical area of focus during menopause.

Symptoms of Cardiovascular Issues

Recognizing the symptoms of cardiovascular issues is vitally important for early intervention and effective management. Chest pain or discomfort is a primary symptom that should never be ignored. This pain can vary from a sharp, stabbing sensation to a dull ache and can radiate to your arms, neck, or jaw. Shortness of breath is another common symptom, often accompanying physical activity or even occurring at rest. Fatigue and dizziness can signal that your heart is not pumping blood as efficiently as it should, leading to decreased oxygen supply to your body. Swelling in the legs or feet, known as edema, can indicate fluid retention due to poor heart function. Awareness of these symptoms and seeking prompt medical attention can make a significant difference in managing your heart health.

Risk Factors and Preventative Measures

Several risk factors can increase your likelihood of developing cardiovascular diseases during menopause. Smoking is a major risk factor that significantly impacts your heart health. The chemicals in tobacco smoke damage your blood vessels, leading to the buildup of plaque and increasing the risk of heart attacks and strokes. A sedentary lifestyle is another critical factor, as lack of physical activity can lead to weight gain, high blood pressure, and elevated cholesterol levels. Family history also plays a role; if your close relatives have had heart disease, your risk is higher. You need to be aware of these risk factors and take proactive steps to mitigate them.

Preventive measures can help you maintain a healthy heart during and after menopause. Adopting a heart-healthy diet is one of the most effective strategies. Focus on consuming various colorful fruits, vegetables, lean proteins, whole grains, and healthy fats. Regular exercise is also necessary for cardiovascular health. Aim for at least 30 minutes a day of moderate-intensity aerobic activity, such as brisk walking, swimming, or cycling. Two or more days a week of strength-training exercises can also help you improve your overall fitness and heart health. Managing stress through mindfulness practices, yoga, or meditation can further support your cardiovascular system. Regular checkups with your healthcare provider are essential for monitoring your heart health and addressing any concerns promptly.

Reflection Section: Assessing Your Cardiovascular Risk

- **Lifestyle habits:** Reflect on your daily activities. Do you smoke or lead a sedentary lifestyle? Start making small changes to improve your heart health.

- **Family history:** Review your family's medical history. Are there instances of heart disease or stroke? Discuss your concerns with your healthcare provider.

- **Symptoms:** Have you experienced chest pain, shortness of breath, or swelling in your lower legs? Keep a journal to track these occurrences, and share them with your doctor.

Understanding the cardiovascular risks associated with menopause empowers you to take proactive steps in maintaining your heart health. By recognizing the impact of hormonal changes, identifying common risks, and implementing preventive measures, you can navigate menopause with greater confidence and well-being. Regular monitoring and collaboration with your healthcare provider are vital to managing your cardiovascular health effectively.

Heart-Healthy Diets for Menopausal Women

Navigating menopause means paying particular attention to what you eat, as your diet directly impacts your heart health. Several vital nutrients play an essential role in supporting cardiovascular health. As discussed previously, Omega-3 fatty acids are important to help reduce triglycerides, lower blood pressure, and decrease the risk of heart disease. These healthy fats help reduce triglycerides, lower blood pressure, and decrease the risk of heart disease. Fiber is another essential component of a heart-healthy diet. Fiber in whole grains, fruits, and vegetables helps lower cholesterol levels and promote digestive health. Foods like oats, apples, and broccoli are excellent sources of dietary fiber. Antioxidants in berries, dark chocolate, and green tea combat oxidative stress and inflammation, which can damage your heart. Including these foods in your diet can offer protective benefits. Potassium, abundant in bananas, sweet potatoes, and spinach, helps regulate blood pressure by balancing the effects of sodium.

Food to Avoid for a Healthy Heart

While incorporating these heart-healthy nutrients into your diet is beneficial, avoiding certain foods that can negatively impact your heart health is equally important. Trans fats, commonly found in fried and processed foods, can raise your LDL cholesterol levels and lower your HDL cholesterol, increasing your risk of heart disease. Excessive salt intake can lead to high blood pressure. Be mindful of added sugars in sugary drinks and desserts; they can contribute to weight gain and increase the risk of developing diabetes, which is closely linked to heart disease. Limiting red and processed meats is also advisable, as they can be high in unhealthy fats and sodium. Instead, focus on lean proteins and plant-based options to support your heart health.

Planning heart-healthy meals doesn't have to be complicated. Start by incorporating various colorful fruits and vegetables into your diet. These foods are rich in vitamins, minerals, and antioxidants that support overall health. Choose lean proteins like chicken and fish and plant-based options like beans and lentils. These proteins provide essential nutrients without the added fats found in red meats. Healthy fats, such as olive oil and avocado, can enhance the flavor of your meals while providing heart-healthy unsaturated fats. Use herbs and spices for flavor instead of salt to reduce sodium intake. Herbs such as basil, oregano, and rosemary can add depth to your dishes without compromising your heart health.

Three Heart-Healthy Meal Ideas

Here are a few sample recipes that are easy to prepare and beneficial for your heart. Grilled salmon with quinoa and steamed vegetables is a nutrient-rich meal that provides Omega-3 fatty acids, protein, and fiber. To prepare, season the salmon with a bit of olive oil, lemon juice, and your favorite herbs, then grill until cooked through. Serve it with a side of quinoa and steamed vegetables like broccoli and carrots for a balanced, heart-healthy dinner. Another simple yet nutritious option is a spinach-and-berry smoothie with chia seeds. Blend fresh spinach with a mix of berries, a tablespoon of chia seeds, and low-fat yogurt for a refreshing, antioxidant-packed breakfast or snack. Try a Mediterranean chickpea salad with olive oil and lemon dressing for a light and flavorful lunch. In a bowl, combine chickpeas, cherry tomatoes, cucumbers, red onions, and olives. Top with olive oil, lemon juice, garlic, and herbs for a satisfying and heart-healthy meal.

Incorporating these dietary changes can significantly improve your heart health during menopause. Focusing on nutrient-rich foods, avoiding harmful ingredients, and planning balanced meals can support your cardiovascular system and enhance your overall well-being.

Exercise for Cardiovascular Health

Exercise is critical for maintaining cardiovascular health, especially during menopause. Various types of cardiovascular exercises can offer significant benefits. Exercises such as walking, cycling, and swimming are excellent for improving heart health. You can walk almost anywhere, making it convenient if you have limited exercise options. Cycling on a stationary bike or outdoors gets your heart pumping and provides a low-impact workout. Swimming is another excellent choice, offering a full-body workout without putting strain on your joints. These activities improve your heart's ability to pump blood efficiently and help lower blood pressure.

As discussed in Chapter 5, HIIT workouts are another effective way to improve cardiovascular health and take less time than traditional cardio exercises with the same benefits. Dance-based workouts like Zumba can be both fun and effective. These classes combine aerobic exercise with dance moves, making them an enjoyable way to stay active. The rhythmic movements improve coordination and cardiovascular health while providing a social outlet.

Water aerobics is an excellent choice for those who prefer low-impact options. Water exercises reduce the impact on your joints while still providing resistance to improve muscle strength and cardiovascular fitness. These classes often include various movements, such as leg lifts, arm swings, and jogging in place, all performed in the water's buoyant environment. Water aerobics can be particularly beneficial if you have arthritis or other joint issues that make high-impact exercises uncomfortable.

Scheduling and Maintaining a Workout Routine

Creating a sustainable exercise routine involves setting realistic and achievable fitness goals. Start by assessing your current fitness level. Then, gradually increase the intensity and duration of your workouts. Aim for a mix of different exercises to keep things exciting and address various aspects of fitness. For example, you might walk on Mondays, take a Zumba class on Wednesdays, and swim on Fridays. Balancing different types of exercises ensures that you work on endurance, strength, and flexibility, all of which are important for overall health.

Scheduling regular workout times can help make exercise a consistent part of your routine. Find a time of day that works best for you and stick to it. Whether you prefer morning, lunchtime, or evening, having a set time for exercise can make it easier to stay committed. Incorporating simple physical activity into your daily life can also be beneficial. Small changes like taking the stairs instead of the elevator or taking short walks during breaks can add up and improve your overall fitness.

Maintaining a regular exercise routine offers numerous cardiovascular benefits. Regular physical activity lowers blood pressure and can help lower cholesterol levels, reducing the risk of heart disease. Exercise improves circulation and arterial health, efficiently delivering oxygen and nutrients to your body's tissues. Regular workouts also enhance overall heart function and endurance, making everyday activities easier and less tiring and significantly reducing the risk of cardiovascular diseases.

Safety is so important when starting a new exercise, especially if you have existing health conditions. Always begin your exercises with a warm-up to prepare your muscles and joints for the activity ahead. Similarly, cooling down after your workout helps your heart rate return to normal gradually and reduces the risk of injury. You need to stay hydrated; dehydration can negatively impact your performance and overall health. Wear appropriate gear, including supportive shoes and comfortable clothing, to ensure you can move freely and safely.

Always consult with a healthcare provider before starting any new exercise program. They can help you determine which types of exercises are safe and appropriate for your specific health conditions. They can also recommend modifications to ensure you can exercise effectively without putting undue strain on your body.

Incorporating various cardiovascular exercises into your routine, setting realistic goals, and taking necessary safety precautions can help you maintain a healthy heart during menopause.

Monitoring Blood Pressure and Cholesterol

Regular monitoring of blood pressure and cholesterol levels is fundamental for maintaining cardiovascular health during menopause. These metrics offer valuable insights into your heart's condition, allowing you to detect early signs of cardiovascular issues before they become severe. Monitoring helps you keep track of changes over time, making it easier to adjust your lifestyle and treatment plans as needed. For instance, if you notice a gradual increase in your blood pressure readings, it may be a signal to re-evaluate your diet, exercise routine, or stress-management techniques. Keeping a detailed record of these readings can also provide your healthcare provider with essential information for making informed decisions about your treatment.

Monitoring your blood pressure at home is straightforward with the right tools and techniques. A home blood pressure monitor can give you a clear picture of your cardiovascular health. To use it correctly:

1. Sit comfortably with your back supported and your feet flat on the floor.

2. Place the cuff on your upper arm, ensuring it's at heart level.

3. Press the start button and remain still and quiet while the machine inflates the cuff and takes the reading.

To get an accurate average, it's a good idea to take multiple readings at different times of the day. Understanding and interpreting these readings is also vital. An ideal blood pressure reading is typically around 120/80 mmHg. Readings consistently above 130/80 mmHg can indicate hypertension, which you should discuss with your healthcare provider.

Home cholesterol-testing kits are also available and can be a convenient way to monitor your cholesterol levels. These kits typically involve a simple finger prick to obtain a small blood sample. The sample is then applied to a test strip, which is inserted into a device that provides a reading of your total cholesterol, LDL cholesterol, HDL cholesterol, and triglycerides. Understanding these results is crucial. A total cholesterol level below 200 mg/dL is considered ideal. LDL cholesterol should be less than 100 mg/dL, while HDL cholesterol should be 60 mg/dL or higher. Elevated LDL or low HDL levels can indicate a higher risk of heart disease, prompting discussions about dietary changes, exercise, or medications.

Interpreting your blood pressure and cholesterol results can help you identify potential concerns and take appropriate actions. For instance, if your blood pressure readings are consistently high, it may be time to consider lifestyle modifications. Reducing sodium intake, increasing physical activity, and managing stress more effectively can lower your blood pressure. Similarly, if your cholesterol levels are outside the normal range, incorporating heart-healthy foods into your diet and exploring medication options with your healthcare provider can be beneficial. Recognizing patterns in your readings can also provide valuable insights. For example, if your blood pressure is higher in the morning, it might be related to stress or poor sleep quality. Addressing these underlying factors can improve your overall cardiovascular health.

Working closely with your healthcare provider is essential for managing cardiovascular health effectively. Regular checkups and screenings allow for early detection of risk factors and interventions, reducing the risk of serious complications. During these visits, discuss your home monitoring results and any symptoms you might be experiencing. Your healthcare provider can help you understand these findings and develop a comprehensive heart health plan tailored to your specific needs. This plan may include lifestyle modifications, dietary recommendations, exercise routines, and medications, if necessary. Open communication with your provider ensures you receive the support and guidance you need to maintain optimal heart health during menopause.

With a solid foundation in cardiovascular health, you are better equipped to face the challenges of menopause. Understanding and managing these risks can significantly improve your quality of life. Next, we'll explore urinary system health, discussing common issues and providing strategies for maintaining urinary health during menopause.

Chapter 9:

Urinary System Health

Have you ever been out shopping with friends, enjoying the day, when suddenly you felt an urgent need to find a restroom? This scenario might sound familiar if you've noticed changes in your urinary habits during menopause. The hormonal shifts that occur in this phase of life can lead to various urinary issues, affecting your daily activities and overall comfort.

Common Urinary Issues During Menopause

Menopause brings hormonal changes that can significantly impact your urinary health, one of the most common being urinary incontinence. This condition affects more than 50% of postmenopausal women, making it a prevalent concern. There are different types of urinary incontinence, each with separate challenges.

Stress Incontinence

Stress incontinence is one of the most common types. It occurs when physical activities like coughing, sneezing, laughing, or exercising put pressure on your bladder, leading to leakage. This type of incontinence can be particularly frustrating as it often happens during everyday activities, making you self-conscious and reluctant to engage in physical exercise or social events.

Urge Incontinence

Urge incontinence, an overactive bladder, is another form. This type of incontinence involves a sudden, strong urge to urinate followed by involuntary urine loss. It can happen anytime, even if your bladder isn't full. The urgency can be overwhelming and lead to accidents if you can't reach a restroom in time. This urgency can severely impact your daily routine and even your sleep, as the urge to urinate can wake you up multiple times during the night.

Mixed Urinary Incontinence

Mixed urinary incontinence is a combination of stress and urge incontinence, meaning you might experience leakage during physical activities and also have a sudden, uncontrollable need to urinate. Managing mixed incontinence can be particularly challenging as it involves addressing multiple symptoms simultaneously.

Frequent Urination

Frequent urination is another issue many women face during menopause. Hormonal changes can increase urinary frequency, making you feel like you constantly need to use the restroom, disrupting your daily life, and significantly impacting your sleep quality. Waking up several times during the night to urinate can leave you feeling exhausted and irritable, which, in turn, affects your overall well-being.

The hormonal changes that cause these urinary issues are primarily due to the decline in estrogen levels. Estrogen plays a pivotal role in maintaining the health of the urinary tract lining. As estrogen levels drop, the lining becomes thinner and more fragile, making it easier for bacteria to thrive. This increased susceptibility to infections can lead to frequent urinary tract infections (UTIs), a common issue for menopausal women.

UTIs

UTIs occur when bacteria enter the urinary tract and multiply, causing symptoms such as a burning sensation during urination, pain or pressure in the lower abdomen, and cloudy or strong-smelling urine. You might also experience a frequent urge to urinate, even if little urine comes out. These symptoms can be uncomfortable and, if left untreated, can lead to more severe health issues.

The decrease in estrogen also affects the vaginal pH, making it more alkaline. This change in pH creates an environment where harmful bacteria can grow more easily, increasing the risk of UTIs. The thinning of the vaginal and urinary tract lining further exacerbates this issue as the natural barriers that protect against infections become less effective.

Recognizing the symptoms of urinary tract issues is important for early intervention and effective treatment. If you experience a burning sensation during urination, pain or pressure in the lower abdomen, cloudy or strong-smelling urine, or a frequent urge to urinate with little output, you need to consult a healthcare provider. Early treatment can prevent an infection from spreading to the kidneys, potentially causing more severe complications.

Reflection Section: Monitoring Urinary Health

- **Daily symptoms journal:**

  - Track daily urinary habits and symptoms.

  - Note any instances of leakage, urgency, or pain during urination.

  - Record fluid intake and any potential triggers, including caffeine and spicy foods.

- **Sleep disruption log:**

  - Keep a log of how often you wake up to urinate at night.

  - Note any patterns or correlations with diet, stress, or physical activity.

- **Consultation preparation:**

  - Prepare a list of symptoms and questions for your healthcare provider.

  - Include details from your journal to provide a thorough overview.

Understanding the common urinary issues during menopause and recognizing the symptoms can help you take proactive steps to manage your urinary health. Regular monitoring and consulting with a healthcare provider can ensure you receive the appropriate treatment and support, allowing you to maintain an active and comfortable lifestyle.

Strengthening the Pelvic Floor

Strengthening pelvic floor muscles is crucial in maintaining urinary health during menopause. These muscles are vital in supporting the bladder and urethra, preventing urinary incontinence, and enhancing pelvic organ support. Think of the pelvic floor as a hammock holding your pelvic organs in place. When these muscles weaken, it can lead to issues like urinary incontinence and pelvic organ prolapse. Strengthening them can significantly impact your overall urinary health and quality of life.

Pelvic floor exercises, known as Kegel exercises, are designed to strengthen these muscles. To perform Kegels correctly, start by identifying the right muscles. One way to do this is by stopping your urine flow midstream the next time you go to the bathroom. The muscles you use to do this are your pelvic floor muscles. Once you've identified them, you can perform Kegels at any time. Sit or lie down comfortably and contract these muscles for three to five seconds. Then relax for the same amount of time. Repeat this ten times, three times a day. Quick flicks are another useful exercise involving rapid, short contractions of the pelvic floor muscles. These exercises can easily be incorporated into your daily routine. For example, you can do them while watching TV, waiting at a red light, or before bed. You'll need to do these consistently to see results, so try to make these exercises a regular part of your day.

The benefits of pelvic floor exercises extend beyond urinary health. Strengthening these muscles can also improve sexual health and function. A strong pelvic floor can enhance arousal and orgasm, making intimate moments more enjoyable. Additionally, these exercises can help reduce pain during intercourse, which can be a common issue during menopause due to vaginal dryness and thinning of tissues. Pelvic floor exercises also contribute to better core stability and posture. A strong pelvic floor supports your lower back and abdominal muscles, helping to reduce back pain and improve posture.

Furthermore, maintaining strong pelvic floor muscles can lower the risk of pelvic organ prolapse. In this condition, the pelvic organs drop from their normal position and push against the vaginal wall. This prolapse can cause discomfort and urinary issues, but regular pelvic floor exercises can help prevent it.

If you find it challenging to perform these exercises correctly or need additional support, seeking professional guidance is a good idea. Consulting a pelvic floor physiotherapist can provide personalized instruction and ensure you do the exercises correctly. These specialists can offer additional exercises and techniques; they might also use biofeedback devices, which provide real-time feedback on muscle activity, helping you understand how to engage your pelvic floor muscles effectively.

Strengthening pelvic floor muscles can significantly improve your urinary health and well-being during menopause. These simple exercises can be done anywhere and offer numerous benefits beyond urinary control. By incorporating them into your daily routine and seeking professional guidance, if needed, you can take proactive steps to maintain your health and enjoy a better quality of life.

Hydration and Urinary Health

Hydration plays a major role in maintaining urinary health during menopause. Proper hydration helps you maintain optimal bladder function by ensuring that your bladder can efficiently store and expel urine. When you're well-hydrated, your urine stays dilute, which reduces the risk of bladder irritation and infections. Staying hydrated is a significant factor in preventing UTIs. Water flushes out bacteria from the urinary tract, reducing the likelihood of infections. Dehydration, on the other hand, can lead to concentrated urine, which irritates the bladder and increases the risk of UTIs. Additionally, adequate hydration supports overall kidney function, helping your body remove waste and toxins efficiently.

Balancing your fluid intake is essential for maintaining good urinary health. Start by aiming to drink enough water throughout the day. The general recommendation is around eight 8-ounce glasses, but this can vary based on your activity level, climate, and individual needs. Ingesting diuretics like caffeine and alcohol can increase urine production and potentially lead to dehydration. While a morning cup of coffee or an occasional glass of wine is fine, try to consume these beverages in moderation. Monitoring the color of your urine can be an easy way to gauge your hydration status. Pale yellow urine usually indicates good hydration, whereas darker urine can indicate that you need to drink more fluids.

Timing your fluid consumption can make a big difference, especially if you wake up frequently at night to urinate. Reducing fluid intake before bed can help minimize nighttime trips to the bathroom. Try to drink most of your fluids earlier in the day and reduce the amount as the evening progresses. Spreading your fluid intake evenly throughout the day can also help you maintain consistent hydration levels without overwhelming your bladder at any one time. This approach supports urinary health and helps prevent dehydration-related issues like headaches and fatigue.

Preferred Beverages for Urinary Health

When it comes to choosing beverages, water should be your primary choice. It's the most effective way to stay hydrated without adding unnecessary calories or irritants to your diet. Herbal teas like chamomile or peppermint are also excellent options as they contribute to your daily fluid intake and have calming properties that can promote relaxation and better sleep. Avoid sugary drinks and sodas, as they can lead to weight gain and do little to support hydration. Sugary beverages can also contribute to urinary tract irritation and other health issues. If plain water is unappealing, try adding a slice of lemon, cucumber, or a few fresh mint leaves to enhance the flavor without adding sugars or calories.

Proper hydration is not just about drinking water; it's also about consuming hydrating foods. Fruits and vegetables such as cucumbers, tomatoes, and watermelon have high water content and can contribute to overall fluid intake. These foods provide essential vitamins and minerals that support overall health. Including them in your diet can help you stay hydrated and maintain a balanced diet, which is particularly important during menopause, when nutritional needs may change.

Hydration Check-in:

- **Daily water goal:** Set a daily water intake goal that matches your needs. Use a reusable water bottle to track your progress.

- **Monitor urine color:** Check the color of your urine throughout the day. Aim for a pale yellow color, adjusting fluid intake as needed.

- **Evening fluids:** Reduce fluid intake in the evening to minimize nighttime urination. Focus on hydrating earlier in the day.

- **Beverage choices:** Prioritize water and herbal teas. Avoid sugary drinks and sodas. Experiment with flavored water using natural ingredients like lemon or cucumber.

- **Hydrating foods:** Incorporate water-rich foods such as cucumbers, tomatoes, and watermelon into your meals and snacks.

Staying hydrated is an easy yet powerful way to support your urinary health during menopause. By paying attention to your fluid intake and making mindful beverage choices, you can maintain optimal bladder function, prevent UTIs, and avoid dehydration-related issues.

Medical Treatments for Urinary Symptoms

Medications can provide significant relief when dealing with persistent or severe urinary symptoms. Anticholinergics are often prescribed for overactive bladder, a condition where you might feel a sudden, intense urge to urinate followed by involuntary leakage. These medications work by blocking the action of acetylcholine, a neurotransmitter that causes the bladder muscles to contract. By reducing these contractions, anticholinergics help decrease the frequency and urgency of urination. While effective, they can have side effects, such as dry mouth, constipation, and blurred vision, so you need to discuss taking these with your healthcare provider.

Another option is estrogen therapy, which can strengthen the urinary tract lining. The decline in estrogen levels during menopause often leads to thinning of the vaginal and urethral tissues, making them more susceptible to irritation and infections. Topical estrogen treatments, such as creams, tablets, or vaginal rings, can help restore the thickness and elasticity of these tissues. These treatments can help reduce the risk of UTIs and alleviate symptoms like urinary urgency and frequency. It's imperative to use these treatments under the guidance of a healthcare provider to ensure safety and effectiveness.

For women experiencing urinary retention, when the bladder doesn't empty completely, alpha-blockers can be beneficial. These medications relax the muscles in the bladder neck, making it easier to urinate. Alpha-blockers are commonly prescribed for this purpose. They can improve urine flow and reduce the sensation of incomplete bladder emptying. As with any medication, discussing potential side effects and monitoring your response to the treatment with your healthcare provider is essential.

Medical Devices for Managing Incontinence

In addition to medications, several medical devices can aid in managing urinary symptoms. Pessaries, for instance, are small, removable devices inserted into the vagina that provide support to the pelvic organs. They are particularly useful for women experiencing pelvic organ prolapse, where the bladder or other pelvic organs drop from their normal position and press against the vaginal walls. Pessaries help reposition these organs, reducing pressure on the bladder and improving urinary control. They come in various shapes and sizes, and a healthcare provider can help determine the best fit for you.

Urethral Inserts

Urethral inserts are another option, especially for managing stress incontinence. These small, disposable devices are inserted into the urethra to prevent urine leakage during coughing or exercising. They act as a barrier, providing immediate and temporary relief from incontinence. These inserts are typically used for short periods, such as during physical activity, and are removed before urination. They offer a practical solution for women who need occasional support for specific activities.

Electrical Stimulation Devices

Electrical stimulation devices can also be effective in strengthening pelvic floor muscles. These devices deliver mild electrical impulses, causing the muscles to contract and strengthen over time. They are often used in conjunction with pelvic floor exercises to enhance muscle tone and improve urinary control. Electrical stimulation can be done in a clinical setting or at home, depending on the device and your healthcare provider's recommendations.

Minimally invasive procedures can offer significant relief for persistent or severe urinary issues. Bladder botulinum toxin injections, commonly referred to as Botox, can be used to treat overactive bladders. Botulinum toxin is injected into the bladder muscle, causing it to relax and reduce the frequency and urgency of urination. The effects typically last several months, and the procedure can be repeated. It's a relatively quick and well-tolerated procedure, making it an attractive option for many women.

Urethral bulking agents, such as collagen or synthetic materials, can also be used to treat stress incontinence. These agents are injected into the urethra to add bulk and support, which helps close the urethra more effectively, preventing urine leakage during physical activities. The procedure is minimally invasive and can be performed in an outpatient setting. While the results can be immediate, they may not be permanent, and repeat injections might be necessary.

Sling Procedures

Sling procedures are another surgical option for stress incontinence. During this procedure, a small strip of synthetic mesh or tissue is placed under the urethra to support and prevent leakage. The sling acts like a hammock, lifting and securing the urethra properly. This procedure has a high success rate and can provide long-lasting relief from incontinence. It's typically performed under local or general anesthesia, and most women can return to normal activities within a few weeks.

It's important to know when to seek medical help for urinary symptoms. If you experience persistent or severe symptoms that interfere with your daily life, it's time to consult a healthcare provider. A urologist or gynecologist can perform diagnostic tests, such as urodynamic studies, to assess bladder function and determine the underlying cause of your symptoms. These tests provide valuable information to guide personalized treatment plans for you.

Exploring personalized treatment plans with your healthcare provider ensures you receive the most appropriate and effective care. Whether it's medications, medical devices, or minimally invasive procedures, there are numerous options available to help you manage urinary symptoms during menopause. Taking proactive steps to address these issues can significantly improve your quality of life and overall well-being.

By understanding the various medical treatments available for urinary symptoms, you can make informed decisions about your health. With the proper support and guidance, you can effectively manage these symptoms and enjoy a more comfortable and fulfilling life.

Chapter 10:

Sexual Health and Intimacy

Intimacy during menopause can be tricky. Maybe you're enjoying a quiet evening at home, your partner by your side, yet you feel a sense of discomfort and unease. The intimacy you once shared seems distant, replaced by a growing concern over changes in your body that you don't fully understand. In this chapter, we will address vaginal health, which leads to some of the most common and distressing symptoms of menopause. By understanding common vaginal health issues and exploring various solutions, you can regain comfort and confidence in your intimate life and enjoy those evenings at home even more.

Vaginal Dryness

Vaginal dryness is one of the most challenging menopausal symptoms. As with so many areas of discomfort you have dealt with, this condition is primarily caused by the decline in estrogen levels, a hormone that plays a vital role in maintaining the health and function of vaginal tissues. As estrogen levels drop, the vaginal walls become thinner and less elastic, leading to a decrease in natural lubrication. These changes can result in discomfort during everyday activities and significantly impact sexual comfort and pleasure. The once-natural process of becoming aroused can feel strained, and intimacy with your partner can become a source of anxiety rather than joy.

Fortunately, several over-the-counter products can provide relief from vaginal dryness. Water-based lubricants are a popular choice because they are gentle and effective as well as they offer immediate moisture, making sexual activity more comfortable. Silicone-based lubricants, on the other hand, tend to last longer and provide a silky-smooth texture, which can be particularly beneficial for extended intimacy. Additionally, pH-restoring vaginal gels can help maintain the natural balance of your vaginal flora, reducing irritation and supporting overall vaginal health. For those who prefer natural remedies, coconut oil is an excellent option. Its moisturizing properties can alleviate dryness and provide a soothing effect, though it is vital to ensure you are not sensitive to it.

In more severe cases, prescription treatments may be necessary to manage vaginal dryness effectively. Vaginal estrogen creams, tablets, and rings are commonly prescribed to address this issue. These treatments work by delivering estrogen directly to the vaginal tissues, helping to restore thickness and elasticity and increasing natural lubrication. Another option is nonhormonal prescription treatments like DHEA, which can improve vaginal health and comfort without the use of estrogen. These treatments are particularly beneficial for women who cannot or prefer not to use hormone therapy. As with any prescription product, please discuss the risks and benefits with your healthcare provider.

In addition to these treatments, several lifestyle adjustments can help you manage vaginal dryness. Staying hydrated by drinking plenty of water throughout the day supports overall moisture levels in your body, including your vaginal tissues. Avoiding irritants like scented soaps, douches, and harsh detergents is also important, as these can exacerbate dryness and irritation. Opt for gentle, fragrance-free products to maintain vaginal health. These simple changes can make a significant difference in your comfort and well-being.

- **Water-based lubricants:** Keep a water-based lubricant handy for immediate relief.

- **Silicone-based lubricants:** Use silicone-based lubricants for longer-lasting moisture.

- **Vaginal gels:** Apply pH-restoring vaginal gels to maintain natural balance.

- **Coconut oil:** Consider coconut oil for a natural, soothing option.

- **Prescription treatments:** Consult your healthcare provider about vaginal estrogen or DHEA.

- **Hydration:** Drink plenty of water to stay hydrated.

- **Gentle products:** Use fragrance-free soaps and avoid douches.

By addressing vaginal dryness through these various methods, you can improve your comfort and enhance your intimate experiences. Understanding and managing this common menopausal symptom can help you feel more confident and connected with your partner.

Bacterial Vaginosis

During menopause, the decline in estrogen levels can cause significant changes in your vaginal microbiome, increasing the risk of bacterial infections such as bacterial vaginosis (BV). Estrogen helps maintain the balance of good bacteria in your vagina, which is essential for keeping harmful bacteria at bay. As estrogen decreases, this balance can be disrupted, leading to an overgrowth of harmful bacteria. Symptoms of BV can be particularly uncomfortable and distressing. You might notice a foul, fishy vaginal odor, which can be especially pronounced after sex. Itching and irritation are also common, making daily activities uncomfortable. Abnormal vaginal discharge, which may appear gray, white, or green, is another hallmark of BV. Additionally, you might experience a burning sensation outside the vaginal area during urination, further complicating your comfort.

If you suspect you have BV, seek a professional diagnosis quickly. A healthcare provider will need to perform specific tests to confirm the presence of bacterial vaginosis. These tests typically involve examining a sample of vaginal discharge under a microscope or testing its pH levels. Once diagnosed, the primary treatment for BV is prescription antibiotics. These medications effectively target the harmful bacteria causing the infection, restoring balance in your vaginal microbiome. Completing the entire course of antibiotics ensures the infection is thoroughly treated, even if symptoms improve before finishing the medication.

Preventing BV is equally important and can be achieved through several lifestyle adjustments. Wearing breathable cotton underwear allows for better air circulation, reducing the warm, moist environment in which harmful bacteria thrive. Sleeping without underwear or constrictive clothing can also help keep the vaginal area dry and less prone to infections. Another step in prevention is maintaining the natural pH balance of your vagina. Over-the-counter pH-restoring vaginal gels can be beneficial in this regard. These gels help maintain an acidic environment in the vagina, which is inhospitable to harmful bacteria. Additionally, using boric acid suppositories can help restore and maintain this balance. Probiotics, whether taken orally or applied vaginally, can also support a healthy vaginal microbiome by promoting the growth of beneficial bacteria.

Daily Prevention Checklist

- **Breathable cotton underwear:** Opt for cotton to reduce moisture and allow air circulation.

- **Sleep without underwear:** Minimize constrictive clothing to keep the vaginal area dry.

- **pH-restoring vaginal gels:** Use these to maintain the natural acidic environment.

- **Boric acid suppositories:** Consider these for restoring vaginal pH balance.

- **Probiotics:** Incorporate probiotics into your routine to support a healthy microbiome.

Understanding the causes and symptoms of BV and adopting preventive measures can significantly reduce your risk of infection. Taking these proactive steps allows you to maintain your vaginal health during menopause.

Yeast Infections

During menopause, the decline in estrogen levels can lead to significant changes in your vaginal microbiome, increasing the risk of yeast infections. Estrogen helps maintain the balance of good and bad bacteria in the vagina. As estrogen levels drop, this balance is disrupted, making it easier for yeast to thrive. Symptoms of a yeast infection can be pretty bothersome; you might experience intense vaginal itching, burning, and redness.

The discomfort can be constant or triggered by activities like urination or intercourse. Additionally, a thick, white vaginal discharge resembling cottage cheese is a common indicator of a yeast infection.

If you suspect a yeast infection, you must seek testing from a medical provider. A healthcare professional will likely perform a pelvic exam and take a sample of vaginal discharge to confirm the presence of yeast. You need an accurate diagnosis for effective treatment. Once diagnosed, treatments for yeast infections are readily available and effective. Antifungal creams and suppositories are commonly used to treat these infections and are applied directly to the affected area, providing targeted relief. In more persistent cases, oral prescription medications like fluconazole may be necessary. These treatments eliminate the yeast, resolve the infection, and alleviate symptoms.

Preventing yeast infections involves several practical steps. Wearing breathable cotton underwear can help keep the vaginal area dry, reducing the environment where yeast can grow. Sleeping without underwear or constrictive clothing improves air circulation and reduces moisture buildup. Maintaining vaginal pH balance is also essential. Using pH-restoring lubricants can help maintain this balance, making the environment less favorable for yeast overgrowth. Over-the-counter boric acid suppositories can be effective in restoring and maintaining this balance. Additionally, incorporating probiotics into your routine, either through supplements or probiotic-rich foods like yogurt, can support a healthy vaginal microbiome by promoting the growth of beneficial bacteria.

Dietary choices can also help prevent yeast infections. Reducing sugar intake is particularly important, as high blood sugar levels can create an environment conducive to yeast growth. Managing diabetes effectively is important for the same reason. High blood sugar levels can lead to recurrent infections, so keeping your blood sugar within a healthy range is essential.

Eating a balanced diet rich in whole foods, vegetables, and lean proteins can support your overall health and reduce the risk of infections.

Understanding the causes and symptoms of yeast infections and adopting preventive measures can significantly reduce your risk. These proactive steps help to maintain your vaginal health during menopause and ensure comfort and well-being.

Enhancing Libido and Sexual Intimacy

Hormonal changes during menopause can significantly impact your libido. As estrogen and testosterone levels decline, you might notice a decrease in sexual desire and arousal. Estrogen is necessary for maintaining vaginal health and lubrication; testosterone plays a role in sexual desire. The reduction of these hormones can lead to diminished libido, making it harder to become aroused and enjoy sexual intimacy. Additionally, psychological factors such as stress and body image concerns can further affect your sexual desire. The emotional toll of menopause, combined with physical changes, can make maintaining a healthy sexual relationship a challenge.

There are several natural ways to boost your libido and enhance sexual intimacy. Regular physical activity is a powerful tool for improving energy and mood. Endorphins released during exercise can elevate your mood and increase your overall sense of well-being. Activities like walking, swimming, or yoga can be particularly beneficial. Stress-management techniques such as yoga and meditation can also play a significant role in enhancing your libido. These practices help reduce stress levels, improve emotional balance, and create a more receptive state of sexual desire. Eating a balanced diet rich in libido-enhancing nutrients is another effective strategy. Foods high in zinc, such as oysters and pumpkin seeds, can support sexual health. Magnesium-rich foods like dark chocolate and leafy greens help relax muscles and improve circulation, enhancing arousal.

Exploring new forms of sexual intimacy can also reignite the spark in your relationship. Trying different types of physical intimacy, such as massage and cuddling, can create a deeper emotional connection with your partner. These activities promote relaxation and build closeness, setting the stage for more satisfying sexual experiences. Experimenting with different forms of stimulation can add excitement and variety to your intimate life. You should prioritize quality time and emotional connection with your partner; set aside time for intimate moments, whether through date nights or quiet evenings at home, which strengthens your bond and can enhance your sexual relationship.

If you find that natural methods are not enough to address libido issues, seeking professional help is important. Consulting a sex therapist or counselor can provide valuable insights and strategies for improving your sexual health. These professionals can help you understand and work through the emotional and psychological aspects of libido changes. Exploring hormone therapy options with your healthcare provider is another avenue to consider. Hormone therapy can help restore hormonal balance and improve sexual desire. Addressing underlying medical conditions that might be contributing to low libido is also essential. Conditions such as thyroid disorders or diabetes can impact sexual desire, and managing these conditions can improve your overall sexual health.

By understanding the hormonal influences on libido and exploring both natural and professional solutions, you can enhance your sexual intimacy and enjoy a fulfilling relationship during menopause.

Communicating With Your Partner About Sexual Health

Working through the complexities of sexual health during menopause can be challenging, but open communication with your partner can make a significant difference. Building trust and understanding is incredibly important; when you openly discuss your needs and experiences, it reduces anxiety and misconceptions. Being honest with each other helps to maintain more meaningful emotional intimacy, allowing you and your partner to explore this tricky subject together. Creating a safe space where both of you feel heard and valued can enhance your connection in ways that go beyond physical intimacy.

Starting this conversation might seem daunting, but choosing a comfortable and private setting can make it easier. Find a time when both of you are relaxed and unlikely to be interrupted. Being honest and specific about your needs and concerns is essential. Use "I" statements to express your feelings without placing blame. For example, saying, "I feel uncomfortable during sex because of vaginal dryness," is more constructive than "You don't understand what I'm going through." This approach helps to communicate your experience while inviting empathy and understanding from your partner.

Keeping the Lines of Communication Open

Common concerns often arise in these discussions, such as the fear of rejection or judgment. It's natural to worry about how your partner will react to changes in your sexual desire or physical comfort. Address these concerns openly. Reassure each other that these changes are a normal part of aging, not a reflection of your relationship's quality. Misunderstandings about changes in sexual desire can also be a hurdle. Explaining that hormonal shifts are influencing your libido can help your partner understand that it's not about a lack of attraction or love. Balancing differing levels of libido requires patience and compromise. Finding a middle ground where both partners feel satisfied and respected is key.

Maintaining an ongoing dialogue about sexual health is just as important as starting the conversation. Regular check-ins and open discussions help to keep the lines of communication open. This continuing dialogue ensures that both partners can voice any new concerns or changes in their needs. Be receptive to feedback and willing to make adjustments. Relationships evolve, as do physical and emotional needs. Celebrating positive experiences and progress, no matter how small, reinforces the bond between you and your partner. Acknowledging and appreciating each other's efforts can turn a challenging period into an opportunity for growth and deeper connection.

Reflection Section: Tips for Effective Communication

- **Choose a comfortable setting:** Ensure privacy and relaxation.

- **Use "I" statements:** Express feelings without blaming.

- **Regular check-ins:** Maintain ongoing dialogue about needs and concerns.

- **Be receptive:** Listen to feedback and make necessary adjustments.

- **Celebrate progress:** Acknowledge and appreciate positive changes and efforts.

Effective communication about sexual health is essential during menopause. It builds a foundation of trust, understanding, and emotional intimacy, enriching your relationship and enhancing your overall well-being.

Medical and Natural Remedies for Sexual Health

Navigating sexual health during menopause often involves a combination of treatments to address the various challenges you might face. Hormonal treatments can be particularly effective in improving sexual health and comfort. Estrogen therapy remains a cornerstone for alleviating vaginal dryness and discomfort. Whether administered through creams, tablets, or rings, estrogen helps restore the vaginal tissues' thickness and elasticity, enhancing natural lubrication and reducing pain during intercourse. For those experiencing a significant drop in libido, testosterone therapy can be beneficial. Testosterone plays a pivotal role in sexual desire, and its supplementation can help restore your interest in sexual activities. In some cases, a combination of estrogen and testosterone therapies can provide comprehensive benefits, addressing both vaginal health and libido.

Nonhormonal Treatments

When hormonal treatments are not suitable or desired, nonhormonal medical treatments offer alternative solutions. Vaginal dilators can help improve comfort and flexibility in the vaginal tissues. These devices help gently stretch the vaginal walls, making sexual activity more comfortable. Another innovative treatment is PRP (Platelet-Rich Plasma) therapy. This therapy involves injecting a concentration of your platelets into the vaginal area to promote tissue regeneration and rejuvenation. PRP therapy can enhance vaginal health, increase lubrication, and improve overall sexual satisfaction. These medical treatments provide options for those seeking relief without the use of hormones.

Natural Remedies

Natural remedies and supplements can also play a significant role in supporting sexual health. Maca root, a plant native to Peru, has gained popularity for its potential benefits in boosting libido. Studies suggest that maca root can enhance sexual desire and improve overall sexual function. Ginseng is another natural aphrodisiac known for its ability to increase energy levels and enhance sexual arousal. L-arginine, an amino acid, is often used to improve blood flow, which can enhance arousal and sexual pleasure. Supplements containing these natural ingredients can be a valuable addition to your sexual health regimen, offering benefits without the side effects associated with some medications.

Holistic Remedies

Holistic approaches to sexual health offer a well-rounded way to enhance your intimate life. Acupuncture, for instance, can help reduce stress and improve libido by balancing your body's energy flow. This ancient practice involves inserting thin needles into specific points on the body to promote relaxation and overall well-being. Mindfulness practices can also enhance sexual pleasure by helping you stay present and fully engaged during intimate moments. Techniques such as deep breathing and guided imagery can reduce anxiety and increase your capacity for pleasure. Integrative therapies that combine conventional treatments with alternative approaches provide a comprehensive strategy for improving sexual health. By addressing both the physical and emotional aspects of intimacy, you can create a more satisfying, fulfilling sexual experience.

Incorporating these medical and natural remedies into your routine can significantly improve your sexual health during menopause. By exploring various options, you can find the right combination of treatments that work for you, enhancing your comfort, desire, and overall satisfaction.

Chapter 11:

Bone Health and

Osteoporosis Prevention

You've probably heard about bone density loss and thought you're too young to worry about such things. But imagine you're walking in your garden, feeling the sun on your face and the earth beneath your feet, when you stumble slightly and feel a sharp pain shoot through your hip. This scenario might seem trivial, but for many women over 50, it can signal something more serious—bone density loss. This chapter looks into understanding why this happens and how to take proactive steps to protect your bones.

Understanding Bone Density Loss

As you navigate menopause, you need to understand the causes of bone density loss. One of the primary culprits is the decline in estrogen levels. Estrogen plays a vital role in maintaining bone health by inhibiting bone resorption—the process in which bone starts to break down and its minerals are released into the bloodstream. When estrogen levels drop, an increase in bone resorption occurs, which leads to decreasing bone formation. This imbalance results in weaker bones, making them more susceptible to fractures.

Aging also has a natural effect on bone density. As you age, the rate of bone resorption outpaces bone formation. This process is inevitable but can be exacerbated by lifestyle factors such as diet and physical activity. A diet low in calcium and vitamin D can hinder your body's ability to maintain strong bones. Similarly, a sedentary lifestyle can contribute to bone loss, as weight-bearing exercises are essential for stimulating bone formation and maintaining bone density.

Symptoms and Diagnosis

Symptoms of bone density loss can be subtle, but you need to be able to recognize them. One of the most common indicators is an increased incidence of fractures, even from minor falls or bumps. You might also notice a gradual height loss over time, often accompanied by a stooped posture or kyphosis, which is the forward curvature of the spine.

Your healthcare provider can use several tools and tests to diagnose bone density loss. One of the most reliable methods is the Dual-energy X-ray absorptiometry (DEXA) scan. This scan measures bone mineral density (BMD) and can help identify osteoporosis or osteopenia (a precursor to osteoporosis). Bone turnover markers in blood tests can also provide insight into the bone resorption and formation rate. A quantitative heel ultrasound can also be used as a preliminary screening tool to assess bone density.

Risk Factors

Various risk factors can increase your susceptibility to bone density loss. Genetic predisposition and a family history of osteoporosis play a significant role. If your mother or grandmother experienced osteoporosis, you might be at a higher risk. Lifestyle choices such as smoking and excessive alcohol consumption can also contribute to bone loss. Smoking interferes with the body's ability to absorb calcium, while excessive alcohol can decrease bone formation and increase the risk of falls. A sedentary lifestyle and a lack of weight-bearing exercises further exacerbate the problem. Nutritional deficiencies, particularly in calcium and vitamin D, are also critical risk factors. Without adequate calcium, your body will break down bone to maintain necessary calcium levels in the blood. Similarly, vitamin D is essential for calcium absorption; without it, even a calcium-rich diet can be insufficient.

By understanding the causes, recognizing the symptoms, and being aware of the risk factors, you can take steps to mitigate these risks and maintain strong bones. Developing a proactive plan for bone health with your healthcare provider might include dietary changes, increased physical activity, and regular bone density screenings to monitor your progress.

Reflection Section: Bone Health Self-Assessment

- **Family history:** Do you have a family history of osteoporosis? Consider genetic factors that might influence your bone density.

- **Lifestyle choices:** Reflect on your diet and physical activity levels. Are you getting enough calcium and vitamin D? Are you engaging in regular weight-bearing exercises?

- **Symptoms:** Have you experienced fractures, height loss, or bone pain? Note these symptoms and discuss them with your healthcare provider.

- **Risk factors:** Consider your smoking and alcohol consumption habits. Can you make changes to reduce your risk of bone density loss?

Taking a proactive approach and addressing these factors can significantly enhance your bone health and reduce the risk of osteoporosis.

Calcium and Vitamin D: Dietary Sources and Supplements

Calcium is pivotal in maintaining strong bones, acting as a building block for bone structure and function. For menopausal women, the daily requirement for calcium is about 1,200 milligrams. This mineral helps maintain the rigidity and density of your bones, ensuring they remain strong. When you don't get enough calcium, your body starts to pull it from your bones to maintain essential bodily functions, leading to weakened bones and an increased risk of fractures. Over time, this deficiency can contribute to osteoporosis, a condition characterized by brittle and fragile bones.

You can incorporate various calcium-rich foods into your diet to meet your daily calcium needs. Dairy products such as milk, cheese, and yogurt are excellent sources of calcium, providing a substantial amount in each serving. If you prefer plant-based options, leafy green vegetables like kale and broccoli also offer good calcium. Fortified foods, such as orange juice and cereals, can help boost your calcium intake, especially if you're not consuming enough dairy. Almonds and tofu are additional sources that can easily be added to your meals, providing variety and ensuring you meet your calcium requirements.

Vitamin D is equally important for bone health as it aids calcium absorption. Without sufficient vitamin D, your body struggles to absorb the calcium you consume, rendering your efforts to increase calcium intake less effective. The daily requirement for vitamin D for menopausal women is about 600–800 international units (IU). A deficiency in vitamin D can lead to decreased bone density, making your bones more susceptible to fractures and other issues.

Sunlight exposure is a natural and effective way to boost vitamin D levels. When exposed to sunlight, your skin synthesizes vitamin D, contributing to your overall levels. However, sunlight exposure might not always be reliable, depending on where you live and which season it is. During these times, dietary sources and supplements become particularly important. Fatty fish, such as salmon, mackerel, and sardines, are rich in vitamin D. Egg yolks and fortified foods, such as milk and orange juice, can also contribute to your daily intake.

Vitamin D supplements can help you bridge the gap when dietary sources aren't enough. There are two main types of vitamin D supplements: D2 (ergocalciferol) and D3 (cholecalciferol). Most experts recommend D3 supplements as they are more effective in raising and maintaining vitamin D levels. Combining vitamin D with calcium supplements is often beneficial to optimize absorption and enhance bone health. Consult with your healthcare provider to determine the correct dosage and ensure you meet your unique needs.

By understanding the role of calcium and vitamin D in bone health and incorporating these nutrients into your diet through food sources and supplements, you can strengthen your bones and reduce the risk of osteoporosis.

Weight-Bearing Exercises for Bone Health

Weight-bearing exercises are vitally important in maintaining bone health, particularly during menopause. These exercises create mechanical stress on your bones, stimulating bone formation and improving bone density and strength. This mechanical stress signals your body to build more bone tissue, making your bones stronger and less prone to fractures. Additionally, weight-bearing exercises help improve your balance and coordination, reducing the risk of falls, which is especially important as bone density decreases with age.

There are various types of weight-bearing exercises you can incorporate into your routine to benefit your bone health. Walking and hiking are excellent options, as they are low-impact yet effective in building bone strength. These activities not only improve your bone density but also enhance cardiovascular health. Running and jogging, despite having a greater impact on your joints, offer even more significant benefits for bone formation due to the increased mechanical stress they place on your bones. Dancing and aerobics can be fun and effective if you enjoy more rhythmic activities. These exercises combine weight-bearing movements with cardiovascular benefits, making them a great addition to your routine. Strength training with weights or resistance bands is another powerful way to build bone density. These exercises specifically target the bones and muscles, helping to maintain and even increase bone mass.

Creating a balanced exercise routine for bone health involves combining weight-bearing exercises with flexibility and balance training. Begin by setting realistic goals that align with your current fitness level. Gradually increase the intensity and duration of your exercises to avoid overexertion and reduce the risk of injury. Consistency and regularity are key to reaping the benefits of these exercises. Aim to incorporate weight-bearing activities into your daily routine. Simple actions like taking the stairs (instead of the elevator) or gardening can add valuable weight-bearing exercise to your day. Gardening, for example, involves lifting, digging, and squatting, contributing to bone health. By making these activities a regular part of your life, you can maintain strong bones without feeling overwhelmed by a strict exercise regimen.

Safety is the most important consideration when engaging in weight-bearing exercises, especially if you have existing bone density issues. Begin each session with a proper warm-up to prepare your muscles and joints for the activity. This warm-up can include light cardio, such as brisk walking or gentle stretching. A cool-down period is equally important to gradually bring your heart rate back to normal and prevent muscle stiffness. Using correct form and technique is pivotal if you want to avoid injuries. If you're new to a particular exercise, consider working with a certified trainer to ensure you're performing the movements correctly. Listen to your body and avoid pushing yourself too hard. If you experience pain or discomfort, take a break and assess whether you need to modify the exercise. It's always wise to consult with your healthcare provider before starting a new exercise program, especially if you have existing health conditions or concerns about your bone density. They can provide personalized recommendations and ensure your exercise routine is safe and effective.

Weight-bearing exercises are powerful in maintaining and improving bone health during menopause. By understanding the benefits, incorporating various exercises, creating a balanced routine, and prioritizing safety, you can strengthen your bones and reduce the risk of osteoporosis.

Medical Treatments for Osteoporosis Prevention

Medications for osteoporosis offer effective ways to prevent and treat bone loss, ensuring your bones remain as strong as possible. Bisphosphonates are the most commonly prescribed medications for osteoporosis prevention. They work by inhibiting osteoclasts, the cells responsible for bone resorption. By reducing the activity of these cells, bisphosphonates help maintain bone density and reduce the risk of fractures. These medications are effective but require careful adherence to dosing instructions to avoid potential side effects such as gastrointestinal discomfort.

Selective estrogen receptor modulators (SERMs) offer another approach by mimicking estrogen's beneficial effects on bone density without some of the risks associated with hormone replacement therapy (HRT). These medications can help you maintain bone mass and reduce the likelihood of vertebral fractures. It's important to discuss with your healthcare provider whether SERMs are a suitable option for you, especially if you have a history of blood clots or stroke.

Parathyroid hormone analogs are another powerful option for treating osteoporosis. These medications stimulate new bone formation by the promotion of osteoblasts, the cells responsible for building bone. They are typically prescribed for individuals at high risk of fractures or those who haven't responded well to other treatments.

Monoclonal antibodies can provide another innovative treatment option. They work by inhibiting a protein involved in the formation and function of osteoclasts, thereby reducing bone resorption. These treatments are administered through injections every six months, offering a convenient alternative to daily or weekly medications. Monoclonal antibodies have been shown to increase bone density and reduce fracture risk effectively.

The Role of HRT

HRT can also play a significant role in preventing osteoporosis by compensating for the decline in estrogen levels during menopause. Estrogen maintains bone density by inhibiting bone resorption. By restoring estrogen levels, HRT can help preserve bone mass and reduce the risk of fractures. However, it's essential to weigh the benefits and risks of HRT—it can be highly effective in maintaining bone health, but it may increase the risk of breast cancer, blood clots, and stroke. You want a personalized approach to HRT, one that considers your individual risk factors and health history. Your healthcare provider can help create a plan that balances the benefits of bone health with potential risks.

Non-pharmacological interventions are equally important in maintaining bone health. Supplements like calcium and vitamin D are foundational. Ensuring you get enough of these nutrients supports bone formation and helps prevent fractures. Maintaining a balanced diet rich in bone-friendly nutrients and engaging in regular physical activity are necessary lifestyle modifications. As discussed earlier, weight-bearing exercises stimulate bone formation and improve bone density. Fall prevention strategies are also crucial in reducing fracture risk. Simple measures like removing tripping hazards, using assistive devices, and ensuring adequate lighting can make a significant difference.

Regular monitoring and follow-up are essential components of osteoporosis prevention. Scheduling regular bone density scans, such as DEXA scans, helps track your bone health over time.

These scans provide valuable information on your bone mineral density and help identify any changes or deterioration. Based on the results, your healthcare provider can adjust your treatment plan as needed to ensure optimal bone health. Working closely with your healthcare provider allows for ongoing assessment and timely interventions, maximizing the effectiveness of your osteoporosis prevention strategy.

By understanding the range of medical treatments available, from medications to non-pharmacological interventions, you can take proactive steps to protect your bone health. Regular monitoring and personalized care are key to navigating this phase of life with strength and confidence.

Chapter 12:

Skin and Hair Changes

Have you ever looked in the mirror and noticed that your skin appears different—more lined, less vibrant, and drier than you remember? Maybe you touched your face and felt a texture that wasn't there before. These changes can be upsetting and are shared by women going through menopause. Like the rest of your body, your skin changes significantly during this phase. Understanding these changes can help you maintain your skin's health and vitality.

Understanding Skin Changes During Menopause

One of the most striking changes during menopause is the impact on your skin. Hormonal fluctuations, particularly the decline in estrogen, play a pivotal role in this transformation. Estrogen is a key hormone in maintaining skin health; it stimulates collagen production, which keeps your skin firm and elastic. As estrogen levels drop, so does collagen production, reducing skin elasticity. This drop in estrogen manifests as sagging skin and the formation of fine lines and deeper wrinkles. Additionally, the skin becomes thinner, making it more susceptible to injury and less capable of retaining moisture.

The decrease in estrogen also affects the skin's natural oil production. Estrogen helps to regulate sebaceous glands, which produce sebum, the oil that keeps your skin moisturized and protected. With lower estrogen levels, these glands produce less oil, leading to increased dryness and a higher risk of irritation. This decrease in oil production can make your skin feel tight, flaky, and more sensitive to environmental factors and skincare products. You might notice that your skin's texture has changed, becoming rougher and less smooth than it used to be.

Several common skin concerns arise during menopause, driven by these hormonal changes. Fine lines and wrinkles become more pronounced, particularly around the eyes, mouth, and forehead. Age spots, also known as hyperpigmentation, may appear or darken due to cumulative sun exposure and hormonal shifts. These spots are patches of skin that become darker than the surrounding areas and are more common as you age. Additionally, dryness and flakiness become persistent issues as the skin struggles to retain moisture. Increased sensitivity and redness are also common, with many women experiencing an uptick in rosacea symptoms, characterized by facial redness, bumps, and visible blood vessels.

The underlying mechanisms behind these skin changes are multifaceted. The loss of skin moisture is a significant factor, as decreased natural oil production compromises the skin barrier and makes it more prone to dehydration. A slower cell turnover rate means dead skin cells accumulate on the surface, leading to dullness and uneven texture. Over the years, exposure to UV rays from the sun also takes its toll, exacerbating the appearance of wrinkles, age spots, and other signs of skin aging.

If left untreated, these skin changes can have long-term effects. Fine lines and wrinkles can deepen, making them more challenging to address later. Age spots may become more pronounced and widespread, affecting your skin's overall appearance. The increased dryness and compromised skin barrier can lead to a heightened risk of skin infections and conditions like eczema, where the skin becomes inflamed, itchy, and cracked. Proactive skin care plays a significant role in mitigating these effects and maintaining healthy skin.

A proactive skincare routine should be customized for you and to the needs of menopausal skin; incorporating gentle, hydrating products can help maintain moisture levels and support the skin barrier. Ingredients like hyaluronic acid, ceramides, and glycerin are particularly beneficial for their hydrating and barrier-supporting properties. Additionally, protecting your skin from further sun damage by using broad-spectrum SPF 30 or higher sunscreen is vital in preventing the worsening of age spots and the formation of new wrinkles.

Reflection Section: Daily Skincare Journal

- **Morning routine:** Note the products you use and how your skin feels afterward.

- **Midday check-in:** Observe any changes in your skin's texture or appearance.

- **Evening routine:** Record your cleansing and moisturizing steps, noting any differences in skin hydration.

- **Weekly reflection:** Summarize any patterns or changes you notice and consider adjustments to your routine.

By understanding the hormonal impacts on your skin and taking steps to address them, you can maintain a healthy, vibrant complexion even through the changes of menopause.

Skincare Routines for Menopausal Skin

When caring for your skin during menopause, the foundation of any routine should begin with proper cleansing. The hormonal changes you're experiencing can make your skin more sensitive and prone to dryness, so choosing gentle, hydrating cleansers is necessary. Look for products free from harsh soaps and alcohol-based ingredients, as these can strip your skin of its natural oils and exacerbate dryness. Instead, opt for cleansers that include soothing ingredients like aloe vera, chamomile, or glycerin. Double cleansing can ensure thorough makeup removal and prevent clogged pores. Start with a makeup remover, such as micellar water, to dissolve makeup and sunscreen, followed by a gentle, water-based cleanser to remove residual impurities. Using lukewarm water when washing your face helps to prevent further dryness and irritation, as hot water can strip away essential moisture.

Moisturizing is another critical step in maintaining healthy skin during menopause. Selecting the right moisturizer can make a significant difference as your skin becomes drier. Look for products containing hyaluronic acid and ceramides. Hyaluronic acid is a powerful humectant that attracts and retains moisture, while ceramides help to restore the skin's barrier function. For nighttime hydration, consider using heavier creams that provide deep moisture and support your skin's repair process while you sleep. Incorporating facial oils, such as rosehip or argan oil, can add an extra layer of nourishment, especially if your skin feels parched. Applying moisturizer on damp skin can help lock in hydration, ensuring your skin remains supple and smooth throughout the day.

The Importance of Sun Protection

Sun protection is non-negotiable. Even if you've been diligent about sun care in the past, you need to ramp up your efforts during menopause. Using a broad-spectrum zinc-based SPF 30 sunscreen daily can help protect your skin from harmful UV rays that exacerbate wrinkles, age spots, and dryness. Avoid chemical-based sunscreens; they can irritate the skin and cause breakouts. Reapply sunscreen every two hours outdoors, especially if you're sweating or swimming. Wearing protective clothing, such as wide-brimmed hats and long sleeves, can provide an extra layer of defense against the sun's damaging effects. Remember, sun protection isn't just for sunny days— UV rays can penetrate clouds and even glass, so daily application is necessary.

Targeted treatments can address specific skin concerns that arise during menopause. Retinoids, derived from vitamin A, are highly effective in reducing fine lines and wrinkles by promoting cell turnover and collagen production. However, they can increase skin sensitivity to UV rays, so pairing them with a thorough sun-protection routine is vital. Vitamin C serums are excellent for brightening the skin and reducing hyperpigmentation. This powerful antioxidant neutralizes free radicals and supports collagen synthesis, giving your skin a more radiant appearance. Peptides are another valuable ingredient, as they help to boost collagen production and improve skin elasticity. Exfoliating acids, such as alpha hydroxy acids (AHAs) and beta hydroxy acids (BHAs), can enhance skin texture by removing dead skin cells and promoting a smoother, more even complexion.

- **Morning routine:** Use a gentle, hydrating cleanser. Apply a moisturizer with hyaluronic acid and ceramides. Don't forget broad-spectrum SPF 30+ sunscreen.

- **Midday:** If you're outdoors, reapply sunscreen. For a hydration boost, carry a facial mist with hyaluronic acid.

- **Evening routine:** Double cleanse if you wear makeup. Use a heavier night cream and consider incorporating facial oils. Apply targeted treatments like retinoids or vitamin C serums.

- **Weekly:** Exfoliate with AHAs or BHAs to improve skin texture and remove dead skin cells.

By following these guidelines and understanding your skin's specific needs during menopause, you can maintain a radiant, healthy complexion even through the changes.

Managing Hair Loss and Thinning Hair

It can be disheartening to notice more hair in your brush or a widening part on your head. Hair loss and thinning are common issues during menopause, driven primarily by hormonal changes. As estrogen and progesterone levels decline, your hair's growth cycle is disrupted. These hormones play a pivotal role in maintaining hair density and growth. Lower levels mean that hair grows more slowly and falls out more quickly.

Additionally, the decrease in estrogen makes your hair follicles more sensitive to androgens, or male hormones, which can cause follicles to shrink and produce finer, thinner hair. Stress and nutritional deficiencies further exacerbate hair loss. Chronic stress elevates cortisol levels, negatively impacting your hair follicles and leading to increased shedding. A diet lacking essential nutrients can weaken hair, making it more prone to breakage and loss.

You can adopt several lifestyle changes to support hair health during menopause. Reducing stress is always hugely important. Incorporating relaxation techniques such as mindfulness meditation, yoga, or simply taking time for activities you enjoy can significantly decrease cortisol levels. Ensuring you get adequate sleep is also integral, as it allows your body to repair and regenerate. Avoiding tight hairstyles that pull on your hair can prevent unnecessary stress on the follicles, reducing the risk of traction alopecia. Limit heat-styling tools and chemical treatments, which can weaken hair and lead to breakage. Embrace air drying and use nourishing hair masks to keep your hair strong and healthy.

Topical Treatments and Medical Interventions for Hair Loss

Topical treatments can also be highly effective in managing hair loss. Minoxidil is a popular over-the-counter treatment that can stimulate hair growth. It works by prolonging the growth phase of hair follicles and increasing blood flow to the scalp. Applying it twice daily can yield noticeable results over several months. Essential oils such as rosemary and peppermint oil have also been found to promote hair growth by increasing blood flow to the scalp and reducing inflammation. These oils can be diluted with carrier oil and massaged into the scalp to improve circulation and stimulate follicles. Regular scalp massages can enhance blood circulation, delivering more nutrients to hair follicles and promoting healthier growth.

For severe hair loss, medical interventions may be necessary. Prescription medications like finasteride, typically used under medical supervision, can help by blocking the hormone DHT, which is responsible for hair follicle shrinkage. Platelet-rich plasma (PRP) therapy is another option. This treatment involves drawing a small amount of your blood, processing it to concentrate the platelets, and injecting the platelet-rich plasma into your scalp to stimulate hair growth. Hair-transplant surgery is a more invasive option but can provide permanent results by transplanting hair follicles from one part of your scalp to thinning areas. Consulting a dermatologist or trichologist can provide personalized treatment plans.

Incorporating these strategies into your daily routine can help you manage hair loss and maintain hair health during menopause.

Nutritional Supplements for Skin and Hair Health

As you navigate the changes that come with menopause, you might find that your skin and hair need more support than they once did. Nutritional supplements can play a significant role in maintaining their health and vitality. One key nutrient for hair strength and growth is biotin, also known as vitamin B7. Biotin supports the production of keratin, a protein that forms the structure of hair, nails, and skin. Including biotin in your diet can help reduce hair thinning and promote stronger, healthier hair.

Vitamin E is another effective nutrient that benefits both your skin and hair. Known for its antioxidant properties, vitamin E helps repair damaged skin cells and provides hydration, reducing the appearance of fine lines and wrinkles. It also supports scalp health, which is essential for hair growth. Omega-3 fatty acids are vital for reducing inflammation in the body, including the skin and scalp. These healthy fats can help keep your skin hydrated and supple while promoting a healthy scalp environment supporting hair growth. Zinc is essential for skin healing and maintaining the strength of hair follicles. It plays a critical role in protein synthesis and cell division, and it is vital for skin repair and hair growth.

How Diet and Supplements Can Help

Incorporating foods rich in these essential nutrients into your diet can make a noticeable difference in your skin and hair health. Eggs and nuts are excellent sources of biotin, and they are easy to incorporate into your meals, whether you enjoy them for breakfast or as a snack. Leafy greens and seeds, such as spinach and sunflower seeds, are packed with vitamin E. Adding a handful of nuts or seeds to your salads or smoothies can boost your intake of this important nutrient. Fatty fish like salmon and mackerel are rich in Omega-3s. These fish are delicious and provide the healthy fats that keep your skin and hair looking their best. Meat and legumes, such as beef, chicken, lentils, and chickpeas, are excellent sources of zinc. These foods can easily be included in your main meals to ensure you get enough of this essential mineral.

Choosing the right supplements can also support your skin and hair health. Multivitamins explicitly formulated for skin and hair health often contain a balanced mix of vitamins and minerals that target your needs during menopause. Look for supplements with biotin, vitamin E, Omega-3 fatty acids, and zinc. Collagen supplements are another excellent option.

Collagen is a protein that gives your skin its elasticity and strength. As you age, collagen production decreases, leading to sagging skin and wrinkles. A collagen supplement can help support your skin's elasticity and reduce the signs of aging. Before starting any new supplement, it's always a good idea to consult with a healthcare provider. They can help you determine the correct dosage and ensure the supplements won't interact with any medications you may be taking.

Consistency and monitoring are key to seeing results from nutritional supplements. It's important to take your supplements regularly as directed; skipping doses can reduce their effectiveness. Keep track of any improvements in your skin and hair condition. You might notice that your skin feels more hydrated or that your hair looks shinier and fuller. If you don't see any improvement after a few months, it may be worth adjusting the dosage or trying a different supplement. Sometimes, finding what works best for you takes trial and error. Seek professional advice if you have any concerns or don't see results. A healthcare provider can help you adjust your regimen to better suit your needs.

Understanding the impact of nutritional supplements on your skin and hair health is an important aspect of managing menopause. By incorporating essential nutrients into your diet and choosing the right supplements, you can support your body's needs during this transitional phase. Regular monitoring and consistency will help you achieve the best results, ensuring your skin and hair remain healthy and vibrant.

Conclusion

As we conclude *The Whole-Body Menopause Guide*, I want to take a moment to reflect on what we've shared and learned. My goal was to provide you with a comprehensive guide to understanding and managing menopause. We explored holistic and medical-based approaches to empower you with the knowledge and tools needed to navigate this pivotal phase of life.

Understanding the stages of menopause and the accompanying hormonal changes is crucial. By recognizing what your body is going through, you can better manage symptoms and maintain balance. We dove into actionable strategies for managing hot flashes, night sweats, sleep disturbances, and weight gain. These practical tips will help you regain control and improve your quality of life.

Emotional and mental well-being is just as important as physical health. Coping with mood swings and anxiety requires a compassionate approach. Techniques like mindfulness, exercise, and CBT can significantly impact your well-being. Remember, it's okay to seek professional help when needed.

We also emphasized the importance of maintaining cardiovascular, digestive, urinary, sexual, bone, skin, and hair health during menopause. Each body system plays a vital role in your overall health, and taking care of these aspects ensures that you stay strong and healthy.

HRT was another key topic. We discussed its benefits and risks, helping you make informed decisions. HRT can be a valuable tool in managing symptoms, but be sure to consult a healthcare provider to ensure your needs are met.

Menopause is a natural phase of life. With the proper knowledge and tools, you can manage it effectively. A holistic approach—combining diet, exercise, lifestyle changes, and medical treatments—can significantly improve your quality of life. Empower yourself to take control of your health. Advocate for yourself in healthcare settings. Your voice matters.

Incorporate the practical advice and strategies in each chapter into your daily routine. Actively implement these tips to see real changes. Don't hesitate to seek professional medical advice and personalized treatment plans. Your health is unique, and a customized approach is often the most effective.

Join or create support networks. Sharing experiences and supporting one another can make a world of difference. Continue educating yourself about menopause. Stay updated with the latest research and resources. Knowledge is power, and staying informed empowers you to make the best decisions for your health.

You are not alone on this journey. Many women have successfully managed menopause with the right support and information. You have the strength and resilience to thrive during this phase of life. Embrace this time as an opportunity for growth and self-care.

Thank you for taking the time to invest in your health and well-being by reading this book. Your commitment to understanding and managing menopause is commendable.

On a personal note, writing this book has been an extremely fulfilling experience for me. As someone who has walked this path and faced the challenges of premature menopause, I understand the struggles. My hope is that this book serves as a helpful guide and a source of support and knowledge for you.

Thank you for allowing me to share my knowledge and experiences with you. I am honored to be a part of your journey toward a healthier, more balanced life. Remember, you have the power to thrive during menopause. Embrace this time with confidence and compassion. You are stronger than you know.

By leaving your honest opinion of WHOLE BODY MENOPAUSE GUIDE on Amazon, you'll be helping other women find the support and knowledge they need to thrive during this stage of life. Your words could be the guidance someone else is looking for.

Thank you for making a difference!

With gratitude and support,

Michele Altobello, BSN, RN, AMB-BC

References

American Journal of Clinical Nutrition. (2021). *Calorie shifting diets and their effect on body composition and metabolic flexibility.*

American College of Sports Medicine. (2022). *The impact of high-intensity interval training on cardiovascular health.*

The Better Menopause. (n.d.). *6 natural remedies for menopause sleep problems.* Retrieved from https://thebettermenopause.com/blogs/the-better-gut-community/herbal-remedies-menopause-sleep-problems-insomnia

Bonafide. (n.d.). *How to increase your libido after menopause, naturally.* Retrieved from https://hellobonafide.com/blogs/news/how-to-increase-libido-after-menopause

Brigham and Women's Hospital. (n.d.). *Genitourinary syndrome of menopause (GSM).* Retrieved from https://www.brighamandwomens.org/obgyn/urogynecology/genitourinary-syndrome-menopause

Callaway, E. (2021). Genetic variations could one day help predict timing of menopause. *Nature.* Retrieved from https://www.nature.com/articles/d41586-021-02128-y

Endocrine Society. (n.d.). *Menopause and bone loss.* Retrieved from https://www.endocrine.org/patient-engagement/endocrine-library/menopause-and-bone-loss

Everyday Health. (n.d.). *Kegel exercises for menopause: Benefits and techniques.* Retrieved from https://www.everydayhealth.com/menopause/kegels-for-menopause-benefits/

Fein, D. (n.d.). *How bioidentical hormone replacement therapy is tailored to you.* Retrieved from https://www.drdavidfein.com/personalized-wellness-how-bioidentical-hormone-replacement-therapy-is-tailored-to-you/

Georgetown University. (2024). *A guide to perimenopause, menopause, and postmenopause.* Retrieved from https://online.nursing.georgetown.edu/blog/a-guide-to-perimenopause-menopause-and-postmenopause/

Greenfieldboyce, N. (2024, May 1). *Hormones for menopause are safe, study finds.* NPR. Retrieved from https://www.npr.org/sections/health-shots/2024/05/01/1248525256/hormones-menopause-hormone-therapy-hot-flashes

Harley Street at Home. (n.d.). *The importance of hydration in menopause.* Retrieved from https://www.harleystathome.com/blog/the-importance-of-hydration-in-menopause

Harvard Health. (2023). *The benefits of HIIT for women over 50: Weight loss, bone health, and beyond.*

Healthline. (n.d.). *Menopause diet: How what you eat affects your symptoms.* Retrieved from https://www.healthline.com/nutrition/menopause-diet

Healthline. (n.d.). *Menopause skin care tips from expert dermatologists.* Retrieved from https://www.healthline.com/health/beauty-skin-care/dermatologists-share-skin-care-tips-for-menopause-and-beyond

Healthline. (2023). *How menopause affects metabolism and weight gain.* Retrieved from Healthline.

Hot Flash Health. (n.d.). *Exploring the influence of menopause on sleep quality: Symptoms, causes, and effects.* Retrieved from https://hotflashhealth.com/resource/exploring-the-influence-of-menopause-on-sleep-quality-symptoms-causes-and-effects

Journal of the Academy of Nutrition and Dietetics. (2022). *Metabolic confusion: A review of calorie cycling and its effects on metabolism.*

Journal of Strength and Conditioning Research. (2022). *HIIT workouts for post-menopausal women: Fat loss and muscle preservation.*

Latte Lounge. (n.d.). *Nutrition for good gut health in menopause.* Retrieved from https://www.lattelounge.co.uk/nutrition-for-good-gut-health-in-menopause/

Mayo Clinic. (n.d.). *Bioidentical hormones: Are they safer?* Retrieved from https://www.mayoclinic.org/diseases-conditions/menopause/expert-answers/bioidentical-hormones/faq-20058460

Mayo Clinic. (n.d.). *Exercising with osteoporosis: Stay active the safe way.* Retrieved from https://www.mayoclinic.org/diseases-conditions/osteoporosis/in-depth/osteoporosis/art-20044989

Mayo Clinic. (n.d.). *Hormone therapy: Is it right for you?* Retrieved from https://www.mayoclinic.org/diseases-conditions/menopause/in-depth/hormone-therapy/art-20046372

Mayo Clinic. (2024). *Hot flashes - Diagnosis & treatment.* Retrieved from https://www.mayoclinic.org/diseases-conditions/hot-flashes/diagnosis-treatment/drc-20352795

Mayo Clinic. (2024). *Lifestyle changes to manage menopause symptoms*. Retrieved from https://newsnetwork.mayoclinic.org/ discussion/mayo-clinic-minute-lifestyle-changes-to-manage-menopause-symptoms/

Mayo Clinic. (n.d.). *Mindfulness may ease menopausal symptoms*. Retrieved from https://newsnetwork.mayoclinic.org/ discussion/mindfulness-may-ease-menopausal-symptoms/

Mayo Clinic. (n.d.). *Vaginal dryness after menopause: How to treat it?* Retrieved from https://www.mayoclinic.org/diseases-conditions/menopause/expert-answers/vaginal-dryness/faq-20115086

Mayo Clinic. (2022). *Weight gain during menopause: Causes and management*.

Medical News Today. (n.d.). *10 of the best sheets for night sweats*. Retrieved from https://www.medicalnewstoday.com/ articles/best-sheets-for-night-sweats

Menopause Journal. (2021). *Exercise and menopause: A focus on HIIT and its benefits*.

National Center for Biotechnology Information. (n.d.). *Calcium and vitamin D in postmenopausal women*. PMC. Retrieved from https://www.ncbi.nlm.nih.gov/ pmc/articles/PMC4046613/

National Center for Biotechnology Information. (n.d.). *Cardiovascular benefits of exercise training in menopause. PMC.* Retrieved from https://www.ncbi.nlm.nih.gov/pmc/articles/PMC6163560/

National Center for Biotechnology Information. (n.d.). *Cognitive behavioral therapy for insomnia (CBT-I): A primer. PMC.* Retrieved from https://www.ncbi.nlm.nih.gov/pmc/articles/PMC10002474/

National Center for Biotechnology Information. (n.d.). *Energy metabolism changes and dysregulated lipid metabolism in menopause. PMC.* Retrieved from https://www.ncbi.nlm.nih.gov/pmc/articles/PMC8704126/

National Center for Biotechnology Information. (n.d.). *Local effects of vaginally administered estrogen therapy. PMC.* Retrieved from https://www.ncbi.nlm.nih.gov/pmc/articles/PMC3252029/

National Center for Biotechnology Information. (n.d.). *Menopause and women's cardiovascular health: Is it really impacted? PMC.* Retrieved from https://www.ncbi.nlm.nih.gov/pmc/articles/PMC10074318/

National Center for Biotechnology Information. (n.d.). *Obstructive sleep apnea: Women's perspective.* PMC. Retrieved from https://www.ncbi.nlm.nih.gov/pmc/articles/PMC5323064/

National Center for Biotechnology Information. (n.d.). *Perimenopause and first-onset mood disorders: A closer look.* PMC. Retrieved from https://www.ncbi.nlm.nih.gov/pmc/articles/PMC8475932/

National Center for Biotechnology Information. (n.d.). *Probiotics and prebiotics: Any role in menopause-related health issues?* PMC. Retrieved from https://www.ncbi.nlm.nih.gov/pmc/articles/PMC9974675/

National Center for Biotechnology Information. (n.d.). *Resistance training alters body composition in middle-aged women.* PMC. Retrieved from https://www.ncbi.nlm.nih.gov/pmc/articles/PMC10559623/

National Center for Biotechnology Information. (n.d.). *Sleep disorders in postmenopausal women.* PMC. Retrieved from https://www.ncbi.nlm.nih.gov/pmc/articles/PMC4621258/

National Center for Biotechnology Information. (n.d.). *Urinary incontinence in postmenopausal women — causes, diagnosis, and treatment.* PMC. Retrieved from https://www.ncbi.nlm.nih.gov/pmc/articles/PMC6528037/

National Center for Biotechnology Information. (n.d.). *Wrinkle reduction in post-menopausal women consuming a specific supplement.* PMC. Retrieved from https://www.ncbi.nlm.nih.gov/pmc/articles/PMC4265247/

Orlando Health. (n.d.). *Digestive problems? Menopause might be to blame.* Retrieved from https://www.orlandohealth.com/content-hub/digestive-problems-menopause-might-be-to-blame/

Physicians Committee for Responsible Medicine. (n.d.). *Fighting hot flashes with diet.* Retrieved from https://www.pcrm.org/clinical-research/fighting-hot-flashes-with-diet

PubMed. (n.d.). *Cognitive behavioral therapy for menopausal symptoms.* Retrieved from https://pubmed.ncbi.nlm.nih.gov/32627593/

PubMed. (n.d.). *Weight loss response to semaglutide in postmenopausal women.* Retrieved from https://pubmed.ncbi.nlm.nih.gov/38446869/

ReachOut Australia. (n.d.). *How to talk about sexual health with a partner.* Retrieved from https://au.reachout.com/relationships/sex/how-to-talk-about-sexual-health

Roth, J. A., Etzioni, R., Waters, T. M., Pettinger, M., Rossouw, J. E., Anderson, G. L., Chlebowski, R. T., Manson, J. E., Hlatky, M., Johnson, K. C., & Ramsey, S. D. (2014). Economic return from the Women's Health Initiative estrogen plus progestin clinical trial: a modeling study. Annals of internal medicine, 160(9), 594–602. https://doi.org/10.7326/M13-2348

ScienceDirect. (n.d.). *Bone health and menopause: Osteoporosis prevention and treatment.* Retrieved from https://www.sciencedirect.com/science/article/abs/pii/S1521690X23000568

Stuenkel CA, Manson JE. Compounded Bioidentical Hormone Therapy: The National Academies Weigh In. JAMA Intern Med. 2021;181(3):370–371. doi:10.1001/jamainternmed.2020.7232

Vanderbilt University Medical Center. (2023, February 23). *Study sheds new light on hormone therapy as menopause treatment.* Retrieved from https://news.vumc.org/2023/02/23/study-sheds-new-light-on-hormone-therapy-as-menopause-treatment/

Verywell Health. (n.d.). *Can hair loss be a symptom of menopause?* Retrieved from https://www.verywellhealth.com/menopause-hair-loss-5218350

WebMD. (n.d.). *Natural treatments for menopause symptoms.* Retrieved from https://www.webmd.com/menopause/menopause-natural-treatments

Weill Cornell Medicine. (2024, June). *Scans show brain's estrogen activity changes during menopause.* Retrieved from https://news.weill.cornell.edu/news/2024/06/scans-show-brains-estrogen-activity-changes-during-menopause

Womaness. (n.d.). *7 nutrients for healthy hair, skin, & nails in menopause.* Retrieved from https://womaness.com/blogs/blog/7-nutrients-for-healthy-hair-skin-and-nails-in-menopause

Made in the USA
Monee, IL
02 April 2025